HEALING PROMISES: A PERSONAL GUIDE TO HEALTH AND HEALING

Go tell what things you have seen and heard: How The Blind Sees, The Lame Walk, The Lepers Are Cleansed, The Deaf Hear, The Dead Are Raised, and to the poor the Gospel is preached.

COPYRIGHT

Hello and welcome to another book by André Cronje
Published by Paris France Mission

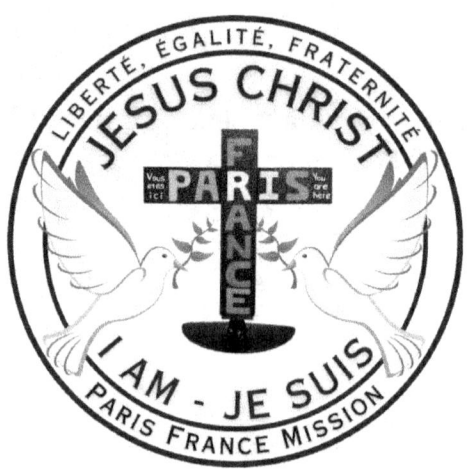

Conceptual Art by André
@shineandre © 2025
In honor of King James

CONTENT

Healing Promises: A personal Guide To Health And Healing

Copyright

CONTENT

1. THE DOCTOR'S REPORT

2. HEALING IN THE POST

3. YOU ARE GOING TO DIE

4. CHEER UP!

5. WOMAN WITH AN ISSUE

6. REMEMBER ME

7. DEMON POSSESSED

8. REST IN PEACE

9. THE UNTOLD STORIES OF DEATH

10. LIVE ONCE, DIE TWICE

11. JESUS HEALED THEM ALL

12. GO TELL

13. BARREN BEARS

14. COVID TERROR

15. THE HEALTHY BODY

   1. Healthy Heads

   2. Healthy Faces

   3. Healthy Minds

   4. Healthy Eyes

   5. Healthy Mouths

   6. Healthy Ears

   7. Healthy Hands

   8. Healthy Feet

   9. Healthy Bones

   10. Healthy Hearts

   11. Healthy Age

   12. Healthy Babies

   13. Healthy Souls and Spirits

   14. God's Body

   15. Body Prayer

16. HEALTHY FOODS

17. A PERFECT HEART

18. HEART PROBLEMS

19. DIVINE HEALTH

20. HEALING PROMISES

The Author's Books

1. THE DOCTOR'S REPORT

Sickness can bind you to a bed and add unexpected financial stress to your life. And with a growing list of ailments, the medical industry, now has its own distribution network of happy drugs and cures. So in a world of darkness, who can see the light and the end of taking medicine? The healthy need no physician, but the sick need a doctor. Besides the finest doctors, medical staff, and advances in the medical field, the world still encounters limitations. Though loved and respected by the community, doctors often become the messengers of death or bearers of bad news. "I am sorry to tell you, but it does not look good. There is nothing more we can do. You have limited time left. Get your house in order, for you are going to die". Your own beloved physician is now the bearer of bad news. Shock and disbelief turn to anger. Some discover new passions, while others spend their living days with pleasure. Doctors may have the license to determine that you are terminally ill or chronic for life, but Jesus is still the great physician with the power to heal. God sent his word to heal the sick and dying. So, anyone who is looking for a good report must believe that Christ is God's hope in a sick and dying world.

Doctors do not have the final say on the outcome of life and death issues. The final word comes from God's word directly to you if you want to live and be free from pharmaceutical drugs. If the doctor says, you're going to die, then the response of the word of the Lord to you is, you will live and not die! And if the doctor gave you a 'life sentence' due to a chronic condition, then the Lord declares to you, that his word is Spirit and life and health to all your flesh. Take it daily and begin to live in divine health.

And for those who are suffering from mental stress and disorders, the Lord would say, you have the mind of Christ, "My peace I leave with you". The peace of God dissolves depression caused by worry and satanic oppression to give you peace and a sound mind. Physicians are gifts in God's Health Plan, but Christ is the gift from heaven that healed the sick.

2. HEALING IN THE POST

To you who fear my name, the sun of righteousness will arise with healing in his wings. For God sent his word to heal and deliver the sick and the oppressed of the devil. It is in Exodus that God reveals himself as Jehovah Rapha, the God who heals. And when the Hebrew slaves left Egypt, there was not one feeble person among them. He vowed to be their physician and gave them his medical care. God's promise was one of health and prosperity if they would love and obey him, but they often turned from him to embrace lifeless idols they could see and touch.

One of man's greatest desires is eternal youth, energy, and life. But no matter how much men brew up recipes for longevity, they continue to fall short of eternal life. Doctors provide significant assistance and ease through medical treatments, but many are unable to afford the expensive cost of healthcare. Leaving the desperate impoverished for affordable health care, which Pharma investors looking for profit will not provide. Only the financially well-off have the privilege of having a personal physician. And so the world is divided between those who look to medicine as the answer and others who choose to trust in the healer. Jesus was a man anointed by God to heal the sick. He had no Ph.D., magic, or alternative cures, but he healed the sick and raised the dead by the Spirit of God.

The more Jesus healed, the more the religious leaders felt threatened by this man working miracles. They did not care if people were feeling better. Nor did they care for the things of God. Fewer followers meant less power, less influence, and a smaller paycheck. But Jesus said to his disciples, Go into all the world and preach the gospel to every creature. He who believes and is baptized will be saved, but whoever believes not will be condemned. And these are the signs that will follow those who believe. In the name of Jesus will they cast out devils? They will speak with new tongues. They will take up serpents, and if they drink any deadly thing, it will not hurt them. They will lay hands upon the sick, and they will recover. These were the final instructions of Jesus to his disciples.

The sick, the lame, the blind, the deaf, and the dumb who came to Jesus, all went home healed. They found hope and comfort in the teachings and power of God working through Jesus to touch the sick. His mission was to do the will of his Father. And the will of God was to heal the sick. The power of God manifested through Jesus Christ as he cast demons out of possessed individuals, causing the lame and bedridden to get up and walk while raising the dead, opening blind eyes, and causing the ears of the deaf to hear again. That is the same Jesus crucified at Golgotha, the place of the skull, whom God raised from the dead. O death, where is your sting? The first Adam was the cause of the curse, but Christ, the second Adam, became the remedy and blessing from God. God has sent his word, and Jesus Christ, who is the word that came and healed the sick. His word is medicine to all your flesh which is God's health plan for mankind.

3. YOU ARE GOING TO DIE

A King's crown has many enemies. Betrayals, death threats, assassin bullets, and public opinions, all compete to clean out the Oval Office. But this message came not from the opposition or the king's physician. No, the voice that announced the king's death was a man feared by all the people. Within a split second, the king's guard formed a shield of protection ready with swords and spears. They have a license to kill on sight and to eliminate any hint of a threat against the king or crown from a foe or friend. Still, there is a slight hesitation. For he who spoke by permission was no ordinary man. And his words are feared, and often the final clause on any matter. One can only imagine the shock and fear at the announcement: Get your house in order, you are going to die. It was a sentence of death without the possibility of healing. For when God speaks it is final, and no doctor or medicine can recover or heal a body whose spirit has departed. Talks of health and alternative medicine were over, and so were the king's plans, after hopes of recovery. A spirit of infirmity and death took hold of his body and he was going to die. It was beyond his power or the powers of medicine, doctors, and healers to keep him alive. Still today, people receive the same message of despair from their beloved physicians. "Sorry, there is nothing else I can do for you. Go home and say your goodbyes". Many never leave the hospital bed. Few have the cursed blessing to know in advance that the end is near like an inmate on death row. Each of us will react differently to the shocking news. The hourglass ran out. No more years or another birthday. Go home and prepare to die.

Hezekiah king of Judah was sick, and the prophet of God came to the king's palace to deliver a message straight from God's mouth.

O king, the Lord says, Set your house in order, for you will die and not live. The death note was not sent by text, post, or social media. Nor was it sent by a devious person to assassin the king. No, it was a direct message from the throne room of God to his prophet to give to the king who loved God. But the king's reaction was not your typical response of rage. He did not order the execution of this holy man, nor did he faint thinking of funeral preparation instead of a royal banquet. He did not seek alternative solutions or second opinions from medical experts in their field. No, he was a man who believed and feared the prophets of God even as a king. And so, in the worst moment of his life, and against hope in the hope he believed, the king, then turned facing the wall cried to God, saying, Lord, please remember me, how I have walked before you in truth and with a perfect heart, and have done that which was good in your sight. And he wept bitterly.

And as the king's tears fell onto the marble inside his grand palace, the prophet was about to exit the king's court. At that very moment God spoke again to the prophet, and said, Go back and tell the king, the Lord God of David says, I have heard your prayer and I have seen your tears. See, I will add to your days fifteen more years. Not only will I heal you, but I will also deliver you and this city out of the hand of the king of Assyria to defend this city.

But the king was no fool. He knew God was not confused. Twice the man of God entered into his private chambers but with a conflicting message. The king did not want to be comforted with a false hope. So, he demanded, if God really did change his decision, what would be the sign, that I will live and defeat my enemy? Then the prophet said: Oh king, Do you want God to turn back the shadow of the sun, or fast forward it by 10 degrees? So the king thought the first is to easy and chose the latter. And God did it according to the king's wishes and turned the clock backwards. And not only did God heal the king, but he also delivered the city from their enemies and caused the shadow of the sun to go backwards ten degree's which caused quite a stir in the scientific community around the world. How awesome that God would remember kindness towards this king and the good that the king has done to lengthen his life.

Hezekiah was a good king who served God all his days. He feared God and the man of God, the prophet who announced to him his death sentence. He did not beg the prophet to pray for him, nor did he complain or burst out in anger toward the messenger. No! he turned to the only one who in times past saved and delivered him. Neither was his first response a helpless cry. No! with hope, he declared: God remember me, and he wept. The matter was so urgent and serious that he prayed himself for himself. When Jesus was hanging on the cross between two criminals, I heard the same words spoken by one of them. Lord, remember me when you come into your kingdom. And Jesus' immediate response was: Today, you will be with me in paradise. Wow, wow, wow for those who believe for they will see God face to face in his glory. But woe, woe, woe unto the people who forget God and remember him not, for there is no hope in their end.

In a similar story, another king also became terminally ill. But unlike the previous king, this king ignored God and went to see the finest of doctors he could find. He even consulted a lifeless idol as a form of alternative spiritual healing. So, God sent his prophet to meet with the king's servants and to convey to them the bad report that God said: King Ahaziah, your sickbed will become his deathbed, never to rise again.

The same happened to King Amaziah whom the Lord smote with leprosy and was a chronic patient until his death years later. Even the prophet Elisha became terminally ill and died, but when a dead man was buried on top of his bones, the dead soldier came back to life. Prophets and prophecy carry with them the seeds of life and death. Believe in the prophet and you will prosper. For the word of the Lord, he speaks will be life and health to all your flesh. The word of the Lord will sustain you on your bed of sickness. O death, where is your sting? Did he not say, you will not die, but live to declare the works of the Lord? Jesus told his disciples that Lazarus's sickness was not unto death. Yet he died. But four days later Jesus went to his grave to grieve but also to raise him from the grave in the sight of all the mourners present. He even interrupted funeral processions, and once raised a mother's child back to life, as he turned their mourning into joy and one happy memorial reunion.

But we have the sentence of death in ourselves that we should not trust in ourselves, but in God who raises the dead. 1 Corinthians 1:9

4. CHEER UP!

I have good news for you. Isaiah said the arm of the Lord has been revealed. He grew up before you like a young plant and as a root out of the dry ground. His form of attractiveness was not of beauty and desire. Despised and rejected he became a man of suffering and acquainted with illnesses. You have hidden your face from him, despised and disregarded him. Yet has he borne your sicknesses and carried your sufferings, still you count him stricken, smitten, and afflicted by God. But he was wounded for your transgressions, bruised for your iniquities, punished for your peace, and by his stripes, you were healed. Like sheep, the people went astray and turned to their own ways. Thus God laid on him their iniquity. Oppressed and afflicted, he was like a lamb taken to the slaughter, and as a dumb sheep before her shearers, he did not open his mouth. He was taken from prison and judgment. Who will declare to this generation that he was cut off from the land of the living, because of the transgressions of the people was he stricken? His grave was with the wicked and with the rich in his death, though he did no violence, neither was there any deceit in his mouth. Still, it pleased God to bruise and weaken him and to make his soul an offering for sin. But he will see his seed and prolong his days, and the pleasure of Jehovah will prosper in his hand. And when he sees the labor of his soul he will be satisfied. For by his knowledge, my righteous servant justified many and born their iniquities. Therefore, to him was divided a portion with the great, and he will divide the spoil of the strong. For it is he who poured out his soul unto death, and it was he who was numbered with the transgressors and bore the sin of many while making intercession for the transgressors.

4. CHEER UP!

A man sick with palsy laying on a stretcher bed was brought to Jesus. And when Jesus saw their faith, he said to the sick man, Son, be of good cheer, your sins are forgiven. But the Pharisees watching thought to themselves this is blasphemy. Only God can forgive sins. And when Jesus discerned their thoughts he said, why do you think evil in your hearts? What is easier to say, your sins are forgiven, or get up and walk? But that you may know that the son of man has power on earth to forgive sins; he then said to the sick with the palsy, stand to your feet, pick up your bed, and go home. And immediately, the man stood to his feet, picked up his bed, and went to his home healed. Hallelujah, not only were his sins forgiven, but his body also was made whole. And when the multitudes saw it, they marveled and glorified God who had given such power unto men. And another time, Jesus went to this pool renowned for miracles once a year when an angel came down from heaven to stir the waters. A disabled man was lying there for a long time. When Jesus saw him, he asked him if he wanted to be healed. Of course, he grumbled, but every time the waters started moving, someone else jumped in first, robbing me of my chance to be healed. But Jesus said to him, pick up your bed and go home. Immediately he jumped to his feet, picked up his bed, and went home healed, leaping and praising God for his healing. The waters are stirring when you hear the word of God. And if you are lying sick in bed, or bound in a wheelchair, know this, your sins are forgiven you. You can get up, make your bed, and go home healed in Jesus' name. So be of good cheer and do not fear, for God has sent his word to heal you. Thank God, there is a cure in Christ the Healer. In his name the sick are healed, the dead are raised, the lepers are cleansed, and the oppressed go free.

5. WOMAN WITH AN ISSUE

For twelve years she suffered from a condition that normally would last but only a few days. She had an issue that no man could solve. The best doctors of her day were not able to fix her issue. And like so many desperate people, she spent her entire fortune looking for a cure. But she found no healer or doctor that could restore her health. Then she heard of Jesus of Nazareth, who went around the cities doing good and healing all that were oppressed by the devil. Many believed that God was with him, otherwise he could not do the miracles he did. Her condition forced her into isolation, like so many people today confined to their beds and wheelchairs at home. But she had faith and said, if I could only touch the hem of his garment, I will be made whole. Her heart was alive with hope though limited by her physical and ceremonial condition.

Whether she waited for Jesus to come to her town or whether she decided to go find him is unclear. But when she saw Jesus come to her town, she was watching and praying for an opportunity to slip through the pressing crowd to touch him. And when the moment arrived, she crawled on her hands and knees through the crowd to touch the healer sent from God. And as soon as she stretched out her hand and touched the hem of his garment she felt the power of God entered into her body to make her whole. That very moment, the healing virtue of Christ left him, and she was healed instantaneously from that spirit of infirmity. Jesus himself felt the power of God leaving him. The touch of faith felt different from the touching crowd. Who touched me he said? His disciples thought he was crazy for asking that question. Because the people pressed like rock fans in the hope of a touch from God for their own reasons. And when the woman realized her secret touch became public news, she confessed, It was me Lord. In that moment Jesus became her high priest, as he declared to her, Woman your faith has made you whole.

She was no longer ceremonial unclean and her years of suffering were finally over. Healing returned to her body, and her freedom to socialize with friends and family. She could now join her community and participate in all the activities and normal life. Not only was she healed but she was also forgiven. That is the good news of the gospel. She said it, acted upon her faith and saw the miracle. God wants to restore you too to complete wholeness. This woman was desperate and in her search for a cure, she spent all her money leaving her in debt and in despair. She traveled the world, google searched, and explored every medical option including alternative healing, and acupuncture. Nothing could cure her. Her issue at first seemed small but after years and heaps of medical bills, it became like Mount Everest that left many dead and scarred for life. David said, I lift up my eyes to the hills, from where will come my help? My help comes from the Lord, maker of heaven and the earth. And like so many she would have given up hope, but against all hope in hope she believed despite what the circumstances echoed or the doctor's reports said. She was one of those rare cases that always seemed to relapse after little progress. Options that worked for others did solve her issue. As a result, this caused a huge financial burden in her house, and her loved ones had their share of misery. But she was a persistent and determined woman who would not give up. For if there is a God in heaven, then there must be a cure on earth. It came from the healer who had no medical degree, MD, Pd, or Dr. title, before or after his name and never performed a surgery.

But what was it about this woman that caused her to receive an instant healing after years of suffering and no solutions? How come when she touched she felt the miracle happening in her broken body? Virtue flowed from him to her, and she was instantaneously healed. Of course, she was banned from public places, and in her days, she risked being stoned to death for breaking the ceremonial laws of cleansing. A crowd surrounded Jesus on that day. Everyone was desperate to touch him or to be touched by him. but not everyone who touched him received a miracle. Did everyone who touched Jesus get healed? Everyone he touched got healed. But there were certain places where even Jesus could not perform many miracles because of the people's unbelief. But this woman said All I need is just to touch the hem of his garment. People still today try to touch stars and popes in the hope of transference or a miracle. But when this woman with an issue came and touched him, she withdrew virtue from him like money from a cash machine, and the flow stopped without medicine or surgery. Her faith in him was her deposit that pleased God, who rewarded her for seeking him. Her touch was the touch of faith, which is the substance of the things she hoped for. She got her healing and her health back. The substance that left Jesus' body instantly transformed her issue into a medical wonder. Miracles of God do not come by natural observation. Nor does God blow the trumpet on his glorious works. Jesus healed ten lepers, but only one went back to thank him. Her words stand out as a proclamation of her faith. What she believed she spoke and eventually acted upon. When the angel said to Mary that she was going to have a child and that he would be the Messiah, she wanted to know how it could be. And when he told her, she said: Let it be to me according to the word of the Lord. In Hebrews chapter 11 you can read of men and women who by their faith changed the world, stopped the mouths of lions, received dead loved ones back to life, and many more amazing wonders.

Guard your heart, for out of it flows the issues of life. Some issues are physical, and other issues are either mental, circumstantial, or spiritual. Maybe you too have suffered for many years. You may have gone to many Psychiatrists, Psychologists, or Physicians, looking for health and peace of mind but got no results. You may have even spent a fortune and still have not found good health. My friend, what is your issue? It may be a different issue or not even a health issue but the principle remains the same. You have to go to the one who has the solution to your problem. What Jesus did for this woman he also wants to do for you. He is the healer and redeemer who sets the captives free. Only believe, and fear not. He is the same yesterday, today, and forevermore. This is the same Jesus who was crucified and rose from the dead. Jesus of Nazareth is alive, and the crowds are still pressing to touch him for their own reasons. What will happen when you touch him? Will you be healed like this woman? Declare to yourself what will be when you touch him, or even when he visits your home or local neighborhood. Press through, and touch him with your faith believing for a miracle. His virtue still flows to solve emotional scars, spiritual torments, and physical suffering, for young and old.

6. REMEMBER ME

The private lives of three men turned into a public spectacle after they were sentenced to death for crimes they committed. According to reliable sources, one of the condemned was betrayed by the kiss of a friend despite being as innocent as a lamb. According to the high priest, it was essential that one should die for the saving of a nation. Later the man who claimed to be the son of God would be heard crying: My God, my God, why have you forsaken me, moments before he died? The condemned thief next to him was also heard saying: My Lord, remember me when you come into your Father's kingdom. It was reported that he was loved by his Father in heaven, and the thief who had no credentials or credit worth of praise wanted to be part of this promised kingdom to come. Eyewitnesses have stated that after the death of this prophet teacher, the sky turned black as night for three hours, lasting from midday to 3 pm. The Roman officer overseeing the execution could not help but say, surely this was the son of God.

But there were two thieves hanging on the cross. One on both sides of the one they called, the Christ. The one on the left kept mocking him as if to curse himself to hell. But his partner in crime had an epiphany strongly opposed. We are rotten robbers to the core deserving death, but he has done no one wrong and should have lived. That is why he said: Lord, remember me when you come into your Father's kingdom, and Jesus, with an instant tweet, replied: Today my friend, will you be with me in Paradise. Here this thief confessed with his mouth that Jesus is Lord, and with his heart, he believed the spoken words of Christ. He must have heard the rumors that went viral, how this Jesus of Nazareth, was anointed by God to heal the sick and to preach good news to the poor. But he was too busy living his life of crime. The love of money made him a thief and a fool.

Are you the thief on the left or on the right of Jesus? Many take God's name in vain always saying, oh my God, oh my god, yet they do not know him who gave his only begotten son as ransom for the world he loved. Do not wait till death, you may not have a second chance. What hope in hell will you have then to get out of jail free if you keep rejecting God's salvation man? Hell is forever and has no fire escape. You do not want to go there. Like the thief next to Christ, you too can say: Lord, remember me in your Father's kingdom. For the kingdom of God has come and will be in you. Jesus was a friend of sinners, and he will be your friend too. Whoever believes in him will never die. And even if you die, yet will you live forever?

Heavenly Father, hallowed be your name. Your kingdom comes, and your will be done, on earth as it is in heaven. Give us our daily bread, and forgive us our sins, even as we forgive the sins of others. Lead us not into temptations but deliver us from all evil. For Yours are the kingdom, the glory, the power, the dominion, and blessings forever. Amen.

7. DEMON POSSESSED

Have you seen people possessed by devils? They do crazy things. Sometimes normal people act crazy but that is just because their emotions got the best of them. Demon-possessed people have often been locked away from society especially when they are violent or a threat to society, but still, some roam the streets talking to the spirits that trouble them. Symptoms vary, depending on the number of devils in a person. Jesus would often cast out demons to free people from demonic oppression and possession. One such victim of demonic oppression was extremely aggressive. He was not only running naked like some nudist on a beach, but he also scared travelers on their way to Jerusalem. When the authorities tried to bind him, he would break the chains and run away. He was uncontrollable. But one day Jesus came his way and delivered him from those tormenting spirits. The results were a medical wonder. Because the man came back to his normal self, got dressed, and no longer had to hide in caves away from society.

Then there was this mother whose daughter was demon-possessed. Jesus ignored her and offended her, but still, she would not give up until he gave her the miracle she so desperately wanted for her demon-possessed child. She was not going to give up fighting for her daughter's well-being. She already knew that medically there was no solution. Even the advanced modern technology of this day cannot cure humans possessed by devils. Psychiatrists are powerless to offer any peace of mind to these troubled souls. Some people have found some hope in Priest performing exorcists. Because demons are subject to the name of Jesus and the power of the cross lies in the resurrection of Christ.

Her faith was stirred by what she heard, believing that Jesus could also do the same for her daughter, as he did for that man. So, she searched for him and when she found him, she cried: Lord have mercy on me, son of David, my daughter is harassed by a devil. But Jesus ignored her flat. But she kept begging until the disciples embarrassed asked him to send her away. You see, she was not on the priority list nor on his schedule. His father sent him to the lost sheep of Israel, but she was not Jewish. So, he answered her not a word.

How often have you heard people say, I prayed, but God did not answer my prayer? And so they stopped praying and walked away from God disappointed and angry. But this woman came to him and worshiped him before she brought her urgent request. Lord, help me she cried. And when Jesus said, woman, it is not good to give the children's bread to the dogs, she could have been offended and gone back home fuming at God, and leaving bad reviews to slander Jesus's ministry. She could have lashed out at him for even being sexist by saying, All men are dogs, but instead, she acknowledged that dogs will not share in the riches of God's kingdom. So she answered him, Lord, even the dogs eat the crumbs, which fall from the master's table. And when Jesus heard her response, he said: Woman you have great faith. So be it according to your faith. And immediately her daughter was made whole that very hour. Jesus could just speak a word, and demons would obey. This happened with a military officer whose servant was ill. As a soldier, he understood the spiritual authority and power Jesus had to command whatever he wills, and it would be done. God sent his word to heal and so the officer said: I am not worthy that you should come to my house. But just speak the word, and my servant will be healed. And when Jesus heard it, he marveled at this man's faith and said: I have not found such great faith, in all of Israel.

8. REST IN PEACE

Psalm 23 is the most recognizable passage in the bible quoted by preachers and priests all the time during funerals. Though I go through the valley of the shadow of death, I will fear no evil. Nothing is more feared than death. But for some, it is fashionable to challenge the Reaper for social media likes or some other stupid reason. Some are lucky and get another chance while most die once and then come judgment. And for those left behind, funerals remain a somber reminder of their own frailty. For who can fight with death and come out victorious? Perhaps once, twice, or three times lucky you survive and live to see your grandchildren while the youth never wants to grow old. There are many theories and philosophies about the afterlife but nothing can compare to the words of Jesus Christ where he said: I am the resurrection and the life. He that believes in me, though he was dead shall live again. And whoever lives and believes in me shall never die.

A friend of Jesus became very sick to the point of death, but instead of calling for the doctor, his sisters sent a message to Jesus to come quickly and heal him before it was too late. However, Jesus took his time and did not rush to his dying friend's bed. So on his way, Jesus told his disciples, this sickness is not unto death, but for the glory of God, that the son of God might be glorified through it. He also said to them, Lazarus is sleeping and I go to wake him up. But because they misunderstood him he told them plainly, Lazarus is dead. And when Jesus finally showed up at his friend's place he was dead as he said. It was a terrible disaster. If only Jesus showed up on time his friend would never have died. And he did not even show up for the funeral. It must have been the talk of the town. The sisters of Lazarus had so much faith in him but now grief and sorrow have replaced their hope and the expectancy of joy. Friends from all over gathered to console the two sisters.

Then Jesus went with them and when they came to his grave Jesus wept. It was evident to all the onlookers that Jesus loved him very much. Then Jesus made an odd request. Take away the gravestone. But Martha one of the sisters said, Lord, he is already dead four days now, and the smell of death stinks. But he replied, if you believe you will see the glory of God. And then he looked up to heaven and prayed. Father, I thank you that you hear me. You always listen to my prayer but I say this for the sake of the people here that they may believe. And then he cried out with a loud voice, saying, Lazarus come forth. And Lazarus came out of his grave wrapped in his grave clothes. And many of the Jews that came with them to the grave site believed but some went back to the religious leaders telling them what he had done.

Isn't it sad that when this miracle happened some were overwhelmed with joy and happiness while Satan's offspring wanted him dead and crucified. They love death rather than eternal life. And in the end, they crucified him because their hearts were evil. These were the Pharisees of that day and today twice as dead on the inside talking about God but having no love for Jesus or the truth. They saw and heard of his miracles yet they continued in unbelief rejecting the word of God that came to heal and save them. But God raised Christ from the dead so that whoever believes in him may also live and never die. O Death, where is your sting? O Hades, where is your victory? The sting of death is sin, and the strength of sin is the law. But thanks be to God, who gives you the victory through the Lord Jesus Christ.

9. THE UNTOLD STORIES OF DEATH

Sermons have been preached, ceremonies performed, poems written, stories told, and songs sung to remember the dead. Some thoughts are stranger than fiction but reality proves true what has been believed for centuries. No one wants to talk about death. Life is too short and everyone just wants to be happy. But in reality, death does not care about your happiness. There will come a time not far when even the strong and the brave will cry out for the mountains to fall on them and to hide them from the wrath of God. And during that time people will wish to die but death will hide from them.

But no one wants to die. You have this intense desire in you to want to live. Except for a few chosen whose love for others is greater than life itself. They are our heroes. Soldiers on the front line and those men in blue fighting crime so you can enjoy a happy and crime-free life. Unfortunately, you will hear stories of people committing suicide. Their will to live was stolen from them when they lost their joy and will to overcome the twists and turns this life throws at everyone. Therefore they decided life would be better without them. Sadly, their ill thoughts warped the truth and reality they lived in, and consequently, only passed their pain on to friends and family who did care. No matter the age, or stranger, death still stings.

No one wants to speak ill of the dead no matter how bad some people were. That is because many don't want to disturb the dead. And that is the reason why they always say, R.I.P., rest in peace. Do you really want a wicked person who has done so much evil in this world to rest in peace? Where is the justice then? And if death is the end then what would be the purpose of living a good life?

Not so with the wicked and rebellious always looking for an opportunity to do evil in this world. They don't fear God or death. But they too will die and God will judge every man according to his works. There is life after death and how you live your life on this side of the world does determine where you will spend eternity. Most people die twice. The second death is much worse than the first. The first death is when you die here on earth, and the second death is what the bible describes as the lake of fire and brimstone where those who are judged by God will be tormented forever. You have a choice of your own free will to choose your destination.

When you talk about healing or sickness, death is never far away. You can care less about death until it comes knocking at your door. Your opinions about death also don't matter. Death has its own reality and makes the rules. Oh, you may escape the Ripper once or twice, but he is forever lurking over the souls of men. Perhaps you googled death and found some people died and came back to life. Their stories are sometimes spellbinding and at times hell bounding. That is not a strange phenomenon. The Bible tells us a story of a soldier who died on the battleground, and because there was no time to bury all the dead they through his corps into an open grave nearby. What happened next defies all sense of logic. No sooner did his dead corpse touch the dead bones inside that grave, that he climbed out alive. What happened was his corps landed on the bones of a famous prophet of Israel who performed many miracles for God. Have you never seen dead men walking? Jerusalem has. There was an earthquake and the tombs were opened, and many bodies of the saints who had fallen asleep were raised, and coming out of the tombs after his resurrection they entered the holy city and appeared to many. Death at this moment seems to still have power over men, but the sting of death has been removed when Christ rose from the dead.

Jesus said whoever believes in me will never die. But even if he dies, shall he live? That is because not everyone will die. The Bible talks of the rapture where those who are watching and praying will escape the wrath of God coming on the disobedient sons. The rapture is not a new thing. In Genesis 7:24 Enoch was the first person God took before destroying the world that then was. And in Second Kings chapter two, you will see the prophet Elijah was the second person that never died, for God took him alive into heaven on a chariot of fire. Oh that you be ready. In Acts 2 Jesus himself in the presence of 500 eyewitnesses was taken up into heaven on a cloud. And while they watched him, two men dressed in white garments said to them, this same Jesus which is taken up into heaven will return in the same way. And every eye will see him whom they have pierced and they will weep bitterly.

The second interpretation of RIP is Resurrection In Progress. That is the mystery that remains whom some want to keep hush-hush. Not everyone will experience death. I would not want you to be ignorant concerning their sleep, that you do not sorrow as others who have no hope. For if you believe that Jesus died and rose again, you will see those who sleep in Jesus, God will bring with him. This I say unto you by the word of the Lord, that you who are alive and remain unto the coming of the Lord shall not prevent them which are asleep. For the Lord, himself will descend from heaven with a shout, with the voice of the archangel, and with the trump of God, and the dead in Christ shall be the first to rise. Then those who are alive and remain shall be caught up together with them in the clouds, to meet the Lord in the air and so shall we ever be with the Lord. Therefore comfort one another with these words. For God has not appointed you who to wrath, but to obtain salvation by the Lord Jesus Christ who died for you. So no matter whether you wake or sleep, you should live with him. Jesus said, I go to prepare a place for you, if it was not so I would have told you. I am going but I will return to take you with me. So be ready, Jesus, who defeated death and hell is coming for those who are looking for a better home. I leave you with two songs not to remember the dead but to celebrate the resurrection of the dead. 'All My Tears' and 'Ain't No Grave', performed various artists.

10. LIVE ONCE, DIE TWICE

To live once is not enough, and to die twice is too much. No one wants to die, especially twice. In Paris France, you can get a job in the building industry where men have to die-die before they can go home to rest for the day. Yet those who love these tough jobs wake up every morning to go back to work to die again. This die-die expression can also be found in the bible. Right at the beginning of Genesis, God said to Adam: If you eat of this tree of knowledge of good and evil, you will surely die, die. Still, Adam lived to be 930 years old, before he died. "Die" is mentioned twice here in the Hebrew text. But translators only penned it once. For it is appointed to all men to die once, and thereafter the judgment. But there is a second death, depending on the outcome of your judgment before God. So, everyone dies, but not everyone will die twice.

Can a man really die twice? The first death happens before judgment, and the second death thereafter. Death and hell itself will be cast into the lake of fire, prepared for Satan and all his angels. Death will give up its dead and the sea the same, to appear before the White Throne Judgment Seat of God, where each man will give an account for his works. These men, both great and small, rich, and poor, will appear naked before their Creator and Judge, without a lawyer to defend them, and without a priest to speak well on their behalf. Yes, each man will speak for himself, even the dumb, unless you have Christ as your Advocate and High Priest. And the books will be opened and whosoever name is not found written in the Lambs book of life, will be cast into the lake of fire alive, where they will burn forever, which is the second death. Thus, the second death is far worse than the first. Hell offers no fire escape and the second death is final. But whoever calls upon the name of Jesus will be saved.

A guy called Lazarus had two sisters, Martha, and Mary, who believed in and loved Jesus. Then one day Lazarus became seriously ill and died. Jesus happened to be out of town, doing his Father's business. And even when he received the urgent call, he did not rush back to heal his friend and even missed the funeral. When Jesus finally returned, his friend was already dead and buried for three days. Both sisters were sadly disappointed on his return, and one of them even commented: Lord if you were here, my brother would not have died. True, Jesus said, but he will live again. Yes, I know, at the Resurrection was her reply. But Jesus responded: I am the Resurrection and the life, whoever believes in me will never die, and even if he dies, yet will he live. So, you only live once, without God, but die twice in the end. But if you have died once with Christ, God will give you another life without end. He who believes in me will never die.

Imagine this for a second. People die all the time, but Jesus said you will never die. I tell you a secret not all men will die. For in a twinkling of an eye the dead in Christ will rise incorruptible. Then those who are alive also will be changed and meet the Lord in the air. The bible mentioned two people who never died. One was Enoch who walked with God and then he was no more and the other was the prophet Elijah who was taken into heaven by a chariot of fire. So will it be at the last trumpet when those not appointed for the wrath of God will be taken out of the way followed by the 7-year apocalypse of death and destruction?

Will, you never die, die? Wait a minute Jesus, isn't it appointed for all men to die once? Jesus continued: Even if you should die the first death, you will live again. The second death has no power over the believer who has part of the first resurrection. Beloved, you are blessed if you hear what the Spirit of the Lord is saying to the church. Death is swallowed up in victory. Jesus wept at his friend's grave. After all, he was human too. The loss of a loved one was heartfelt and deep. But then he prayed to his Father in heaven.

Saying, thank you, Father, that you hear me always and that this death is for your glory. So, he told the people standing there with him, to roll away that gravestone. But Lord, his sisters objected: He is dead for three days and smells like death. Yet they obeyed his instruction, for he who spoke creation into being and breathed life into Adam, became flesh stood before them, the word of God, sent from heaven to earth. Lazarus, come out, Jesus shouted! Then silence as eyes stare at the tomb. A gasp went through the crowd as a mummy wrapped in linen came hopping out. Untie him, Jesus commanded. When Jesus raises the dead, they are still bound in their old clothes and in need of a bath and a clean robe of righteousness. Proving to you that no matter how dead and buried your life, dreams, and hopes are, he is able. So, when he asks you as he did to Ezekiel, can these dry bones live again? All you need to do is to believe and say Lord you know, and you will also see his glory. When the crowd saw this, they believed in him and praised God in heaven.

I am he who was dead, Jesus said, but now I am alive. Why do you look for the living among the dead, the angels said to Mary Magdalene at the tomb of Jesus? He is not here, He has risen. And for 40 days after his resurrection, Jesus showed himself alive to his disciples and 500 other eyewitnesses, before he ascended to heaven before their very eyes. Take comfort, he said. I will not leave you as orphans. My Comforter is with you. He will remind you of everything I said. He who died once for the sins of the world now lives forevermore and will never die again. So will you. Death has lost its sting. Christ promised the abundant life, because you believe in him, who died and rose from the dead. He is the living bread, the bread of life.

He was as good as dead but out of him came forth a people as many as the stars in the sky. In Ezekiel 37 God asks you a question. How will you answer him? Can this valley of dry bones live again? Lord you know. Can these dead cells in your body be produced again? Lord you know. Can this bold head be covered with hair again? Lord you know. Can those missing teeth grow again? Lord you know. Can dead rocks sing and praise God when you refuse to dance and sing when the music plays? God knows. Can limbs lost or struck dead by a stroke move again? Lord you know. Can eyes dim and blind see again? Lord you know. He was as good as dead but out of him sprang a multitude like the stars of the heavens.

Have you not heard the story of how they tried to bury a soldier killed in battle in another man's grave? When his body fell onto the bones of another in that grave, the dead soldier came back to life. It just happened that the bones in that grave belonged to a holy man of God Elisha the prophet who had a double portion of Elijah's anointing. And when Elisha fell asleep, he was short of one miracle to that double anointing he asked for. God honored Elisha's request by giving him a double blessing. So is it with a lot of God's people who fall asleep, whose works follow them? It continues to bud and blossom just like Aaron's rod in the ark of the covenant. In the presence of God, there is only light, and the light of Christ is the life of men. So, can these things be? Can a dead marriage blossom with love again? Can dead situations that are impossible with men, be possible to one who believes? Lord you know all things are possible to him who believes. So let it be to me.

11. JESUS HEALED THEM ALL

There was a healer in town named Jesus. Yes, he was Jewish and a carpenter by trade. But when you are sick, you do not care about credentials if someone has the gift of healing. Like that Roman Officer from Italy who came to Jesus and said, my servant is sick and needs healing. God anointed Jesus with the Holy Ghost and with power, and he went to many cities doing good and healing all who were oppressed by the devil because God was with him. He healed the worst of sinners, and he healed the best of saints alike. He even raised his friend Lazarus from the dead. He is Jehovah Rapha, the Lord who heals. Like a man who fixes his house, and a woman her home so is God at work in his creation. But God heals more than just flesh and blood. He heals nations. He heals undrinkable water, and he heals the ground so that it may produce fruit. Look at what God did with the barren land of Israel. There is no such thing as incurable diseases with God. To him who believes all things are possible. Nothing is too hard for God. Jesus said, Only believe and you will see the glory of God. And so, he healed many because they believed.

Jesus went to many places teaching and preaching the gospel of the kingdom while healing all manner of sicknesses and all kinds of diseases. His fame even spread throughout Syria. And they brought to him all the sick that had various diseases and torments, and those possessed with devils, lunatics, and those that had the palsy, and he healed them all. The healthy need no physician, but those who are sick go to a doctor. And if the sickness gets worse, then people start looking for a specialist that would not only tell them what is wrong but also offer them a cure. But if they find no cure, will they still have hope left to believe that God is able and willing to heal them? Come to Jesus and he will heal you. God anointed him for this purpose. Sometimes he will find you lying sick in bed sitting up in your wheelchair or lying down dropped dead in your coffin. Yip, Jesus did find them all, even a demon-possessed man who was always running naked in the hills, scaring travelers and tourists on their way to Jerusalem. But Jesus kicked out those demons that tormented him into the local pig den and when the town council heard that the pigs committed suicide, they came to Jesus begging him to leave. But the crazy man was now found clothed and in his right mind. Unfortunately, the city council was more hung over the loss of their pig farm, than feeling joyful over that lunatic's sweet liberty. His word is medicine to your whole body and nourishment to your bones. He renews your youth like that of an eagle. There is not one word he has spoken that has fallen to the ground that will not bear results. For he watches over his word, which he sends out, to do, and to fulfill it. The Lord is able and willing to do more than what you think possible. You may say that Jesus no longer lives among us. Have you not heard, and did you not read, how after his death on the cross and his resurrection three days later, he continued to show himself alive for forty days, before he ascended to heaven in front of over 500 eyewitnesses? And at his final departure and farewell speech, he said: All power in heaven and earth was given to me to give to you that you may go to teach all nations, baptizing them in the name of the Father, the Son, and the Holy Spirit. Teaching men to observe all things whatever I have commanded you. I am with you always, to the end of the world. And these signs will follow them that believe. In my name they will cast out devils, they will speak in new tongues, they will pick up serpents, and if they drink anything deadly it will not hurt them. They will lay hands on the sick and the sick will recover. And so, after the Lord has spoken to them, he was received up into heaven and now sits on the right hand of God. And so, they went forth and preached everywhere, and the Lord worked with them, confirming the word with signs and wonders following. You live in a broken world that needs constant fixing.

The place in which you live, and work needs healing too. That is why God said: If my people who are called by my name will humble themselves and pray, I will hear and heal their land. Look at Israel, how they blossom and bloom. Once, a desert and deserted land, now covered with fruitful trees and potential. A booming economy means the fat of the land has returned and the sorrow of famine, war, and natural disasters have departed. There is also healing for both the mind and the spirit. A broken spirit before God is precious. But an abused person is like a cracked window. But though the strong may despise the weak, God says come to me, I will be your strength. Many people are ICU cases in need of a good Samaritan to take care of their wounds and to book them into a place of care and recovery. Scars are a dim reminder of past wounds. Whether it be an injury on the playground as a child, or a battle scar defending the land. Nevertheless, some scars came from the words and deeds of loved ones or total strangers. Words that cut like a knife deeper than flesh and bones to lodge themselves in the mental frame of one's soul. And when these wounds are afflicted daily, the abuse affects the person's behavior. Some are lucky to escape its effects, but others continue with the abuse mantel put on them. This will affect how you see and perceive things around you. Sexual assault can be physical or mental. It may have absolutely nothing to do with the other person, as much as their mannerism is perceived as a violation of your intimacy or domination of their private space, even though they never even touched you. Again, I hear the Lord say, bring all your cares, and burdens to him for he cares for you. Your circumstances will not have dominion over you and your past will not be your future. The balm of Gilead will bring healing, restoration, and deliverance from the effects of past and present hurts. Your famine for affection and true love ends when you enter into his presence where there is fullness of joy and healing.

There is no scientific formula for healing the sick. Thank God for your healing, because it is so easily taken for granted to credit medicine or doctors for it. God is at work and will use natural and supernatural ways to bring healing to you. Paul advised Timothy to take a little wine for his constant tummy aches. Coke-Cola helps in my case. Solomon said: Eat honey, my son, for it is good for you. The apostles also recommended that if you are sick, then go to the elders and let them anoint you with oil and pray for your healing. One time Paul prayed over handkerchiefs and when it was laid on the sick, they recovered. On another occasion, he walked by the sick, and when his shadow fell on them, they were instantly healed. Remember the Roman Officer who had great faith. He told Jesus to only speak a word, and that his servant would be healed. His servant was perhaps too sick to come to Jesus, so he approached Jesus on his behalf. He was a man under authority who also exercised authority. And when Jesus saw his faith, he marveled. There was a gentile who was not a Jew, but he had Abraham's faith to receive a miracle from God. Still, some died in hope, believing though not receiving. But God remains faithful. He is both willing and able to do what he promised. He will always be the God who heals. The Bible says that in the new earth, the leaves of the trees will be for the healing of the nations, where death will no longer be. Healing may not always be felt or seen immediately. And because of that, it may be wrongly assumed that healing never took place. While skeptics look for signs, believers will receive them by faith. Let him ask in prayer, believing that he received, and not doubting. Doubt will rob you of a blessing. Why do I say this? After Jesus healed ten lepers, he instructed them to go to the priest to be examined and to verify that they were clean. That was the law before a leper could come back into a community. And as they went in obedience, they were healed. But only one showed gratitude when he went back to thank Jesus for his healing. Did not all get healed, Jesus replied. Sometimes, it's in the action of going to the doctor for a second opinion that you may discover that you were healed when they prayed and laid hands on you. You might even be lying sick in bed, like the great healing evangelist Kenneth Hagin, reading your bible, when faith suddenly enters into his heart to believe, and he got out of bed and was never sick again until his death. Sure, the devil will come up with symptoms like heart pain or shortness of breath and tell you that you are going to die. You can believe the devil, or you can believe God's word. Faith comes by hearing and hearing God's word. Then boldly say, devil, it is written, by his stripes, you are healed. So, take your sickness and disease of me for this body is God's temple. You do not have to live sick for the rest of your life. God's word is a better life companion that will give you joy and peace. Healing comes to those who seek Christ for healing. They may have heard or read how Jesus healed someone else. And because they believe the report they heard, they too can believe God for their own miracle.

How did Jesus heal the sick? God anointed Jesus of Nazareth with the Holy Ghost and with power, who went around doing good and healing all that were oppressed by the devil, for God was with him. They came to him sick and went back home healed. Their faith in him and God made them whole. Often Jesus would only speak a word, and the word of faith would heal the sick. That is how a servant of an Italian officer got healed. The Officer said: Lord just speak a word and my servant will be healed. You do not need to come to my house. Besides, I am not worthy to even receive you into my home. Wow, Jesus marveled. Such great faith have I not seen in all of Israel. Sometimes he would touch the sick, and other times they touched him. His glory was to do the will of the Father, not his own. These signs will follow them that believe he said: In my name, you will heal the sick, cast out devils, and even raise the dead. A few times Jesus interrupted funeral processions to bring back life to the dead and joy to their loved ones. It is the will of God to bring joy into your life. That is what he did for the two sisters of his friend Lazarus when he raised him back to life after he was dead and buried for four days. The Bible is full of miracles and wonders what God has done, and what he will do again for anyone who will believe in his name.

Love compelled him, not money, fame, or power. Jesus was moved with compassion. And when he stood at the grave of his friend Lazarus, he wept bitterly. See how he loved him, they said. Oh, that God would give you such compassion for the sick and needy. Often Jesus would tell people only to believe. Some even cried out, Lord I believe, help me in my unbelief. Faith comes by hearing a message that addresses your needs and circumstances and hearing God's word. But when you hear the negative reports from doctors or someone else, it produces fear and hopelessness, robbing you of faith in a miracle. So shut your eyes and ears from those faith robbers and hold on to his promises for you. And if you believe, then you will see the glory of God. The same works Jesus did, you will do also. For you will receive power when the Holy Ghost comes upon you. And these signs will follow those who believe. They will lay their hands on the sick, and the sick will recover. You will speak to the dead, and they will hear and obey your voice. You can do all these things through Christ who strengthens you. Nothing is impossible to him who believes. It is the power of the Holy Ghost working in and through you. Some have one gift, others have more. And there are different gifts and ministries but all by the same Spirit. There is no limit to the creative ways in which God can use you to work miracles or heal the sick though there are many ways to pray for them. One time, Jesus spat in the dirt and used the clay to form eyes for a blind man. Did not the Lord God form Adam from clay and breathe life into his nostrils? It is not a formula but rather an act of obedience. Remember, even Jesus could not perform many miracles in his hometown because of the people's unbelief. But when he went to neighboring cities many were healed and delivered.

12. GO TELL

Since I became a Christian, I have seen and heard of many healings and miracles. Some of those healings were unusual miracles. Some were healed instantly. We now live in an age of advanced medicine, where doctors are miracle workers until they have to tell their patients, sorry there is nothing else we can do for you. But where hope is dead, miracles come alive. I can tell you from personal experience that God still works today where there is faith. Doubt and unbelief will rob you of a sure miracle. Sin also may have been the cause of some ailments. But because of his mercies, you are not consumed.

Often I would pray for myself, but the Word also encourages us to ask for prayer when we are sick. The church in the name of Jesus has the power to minister healing to the sick. When miracles happen, it is often in such a way that one could easily doubt whether it is God or not. But you live by faith. And God does not blow angel trumpets to announce yet another miracle. That is why it is called signs and wonders. Did he not say that you will lay your hands on the sick and they will recover? That means healing can take place instantaneously or in due process. I remember how someone told me of this guy in the ICU, the doctors said would not make it. After inquiry, I went to visit him and prayed. A few days later I heard that he had recovered and was released from the hospital. On another occasion, I went with a sister from church to visit her brother in the hospital. He suddenly became ill and went into a coma. The doctors could not find what was wrong with him. I remember we prayed together not stopping for an hour. Days later he woke up from his coma and had a full recovery.

One morning around 1 am while sleeping, I was woken up by a

loud bang outside my home. I jumped out of bed and ran to see what had just happened only to arrive at the scene of a horrible motor vehicle accident. It appeared that two vehicles were involved. One was in the middle of the road, and the second was parked in a driveway. To my horror, I discovered that it was only one vehicle, not two cars. The drunk driver lost control and hit a tree at high speed, which tore the car into two halves. The driver was lying behind the front half of the vehicle in the driveway. She lay helpless against the wall, in a half-upright position, and seriously injured. She was heavily breathing gasping for air as blood was running down her lungs. There was no one else to help me. I did not know what to do as I had no medical training. She needed air so I turned her head so she could breathe more freely. Then I saw a big hole in her head where the blood was oozing out. I am no medic, but I held her head in that position with my hands and decided to pray for her. I was praying earnestly for this woman, and I kept saying, Jesus, do not let her die. I rebuked death and declared that she would live in Jesus' name.

The Bible says, whatever you bind on earth will be bound in heaven, and what you lose on earth will be loosed in heaven. By faith we allow God to work in and through us. And faith pleases God. Finally, the ambulance arrived on the scene and the professionally trained personnel took care of the situation. What happened after that I did not know until two weeks later, when someone told me that she heard that this woman was in a coma, at a certain hospital. I was so happy to hear that she did not die and decided to go and visit her. On the same day I went to visit her at the hospital, another miracle happened. She has just woken up from her coma on that very day. Praise God. It was exciting news. I was able to talk to her and shared that what happened to her that morning was a miracle because she could not remember anything. But thanks be to God, she lived.

The most unfortunate thing that can happen to you, is that you are alone when tragedy strikes. This happened to me without warning. I was alone in an apartment when I had a stroke.

I have seen many stroke survivors marred by a sudden stroke from nowhere. In an instant, one-half of my body became lame. Paralyzed with fear, I remained motionless in one position. Without thinking, I started to whisper the name of Jesus, repeatedly. I kept saying his name for about five to fifteen minutes until I felt life restored to my other half. Years later I would suffer a heat stroke and subsequently be hospitalized. Scans revealed scarred tissue on my brain, which alarmed the Neurosurgeon about my health condition. Doctors fervently recommend I stay on medicine for the rest of my life, to prevent another stroke. That was until I read in the bible, how God would heal me of the stroke he afflicted upon me, for my transgressions. I do believe that God can heal anyone, never to suffer another stroke or heart attack again. When you continue to walk and live in obedience to him, his health plan kicks in. When God heals you, you can throw away those labels and medical predictions that say, you are sick for life. I prefer God's label, which says: By his stripes, I am healed. God's health plan for me is to be whole, and not to live in fear of death. I still take some painkillers for the headaches I suffer, but I no longer live in fear. Because I chose to believe God's report as my final health report.

On another occasion, a mother discovered her child lying inside the baby bed not breathing. Startled in hysteria she came running to me for help. I ran to see what I could do. Instinctively I grabbed the child upside down and started to shake him, while I kept saying in the name of Jesus, over and over again. Then the boy showed signs of life, and I gave him back to his mother alive, who rushed him off to the hospital for examination. It always amazes me how miracles never seem like miracles when God does wonders. Often you hear how people died and came back to life. I also heard stories where God would wake up people to pray for a specific person. Just to find out later that at that exact time, something bad had happened, but the person miraculously survived. My dad would come to me many times and say: André, I am dying. But all I knew was the name of Jesus and to pray for him. When people come to me and say, I have pain, I do not often have the faith to pray as I want to. But in a critical situation, I sometimes just jump in and make room for Jesus to bring hope and life. I would always respond to my dad with faith by saying: Dad you not going to die. I did not know, but God used my words to build faith and hope in him to calm his fears. It happened often, and I would always have the same reply and to pray for him. We were poor, and a visit to the doctor was not in our budget. My Dad not only also survived a stroke, but he lived an additional fifteen years in good health before he passed away. I cannot thank God enough.

Did you know that Jesus healed ten lepers and only one came back to thank him? What if you prayed to God for someone you love, and God healed them of cancer, or some disease and you only thanked your doctor but forgot the healer who healed? God uses any available vessel to accomplish his wonders. Sadly, I have seen how some after many prayers still passed away. But the bible speaks of those who died in faith and have not obtained the promises of God. And in trying times like these, when your faith is shaken, keep trusting God. He is the great comforter, and we have this hope that nothing will separate us from the love of God. Neither life nor death, riches, or poverty, or any other thing. Death has lost its sting and he who raised Lazarus from the dead lives forever. The same power that raised Christ from the dead now dwells in you. You are his workmanship created for good works. Anyone can pray for the sick in his name. Some may have the gift of unusual miracles, while others have the gift of healing. But when you are the only one around, know that God will use you to bring glory to his name. Amen.

The Spirit of the Lord is on me because he has anointed me to preach the gospel to the poor. He has sent me to heal the brokenhearted, to preach deliverance to the captives, and recover of sight to the blind, and to set at liberty them that are bruised.

13. BARREN BEARS

Mary was a young woman and a virgin when an angel appeared to her with the surprising news that she was going to have a baby. But how is that possible if I am still a virgin she asked. Then the angel said to her the Holy Spirit would come upon her and that she would give birth to the savior. What is impossible with man is possible with God. So, Mary said let it be to me according to your words. And went to visit her relative Elizabeth who also received a miracle child because she was barren, the child in her leaped for joy when he heard the voice of Mary. Mary was about to deliver God's son and Elizabeth was about to deliver John the Baptist who would be the prophet that would prepare the way for Jesus' ministry. He was calling people to repentance and the sign of their obedience was to be baptized. Jesus himself was baptized by John as a sign of faith. Thus, setting the example to whoever believes in him, to follow him in his baptism of death and they will be raised to life again. The four Gospels

Zacharias and Elizabeth were happily married. And like most couples, they wanted to start a family. But their dreams got crushed after a medical examination revealed that Elizabeth would not be able to have any children. Zacharias petitioned God on behalf of his family, but the years went on, and they both became old. Then one day, as he was performing his temple duty as a priest, an angel appeared to him. Angels often appear to man in two forms. Disguised as a human being which the bible says, some have entertained angels unawares or as angels in their full glory, frightful to behold. In those cases, they would always say, fear not as we would say hello. How many times have Jesus not also said that to you and me? Fear not, I have good news. Your prayer has been answered. It was the angel Gabriel, who stood in the presence of God, with a divine message. He continued to reveal the child's sex, his name, and his destiny to his father. How amazing is that? He said to Jeremiah before I formed you in your mother's womb, I knew you. Out of a barren womb, out of the desert came a prophet who prophesied of another, whose life and words would change the entire world.

From one miracle baby to another super baby. Samson, the world's strongest man was born from the womb of a barren woman. An angel appeared unto her foretelling that she would have a baby blessed by God to save Israel from being slaves to the Philistines. She is never mentioned by name and remains anonymous throughout the whole story. Samson judged Israel until his untimely death, betrayed by Delilah the love of his life.

Then there is Hannah. Her womb was shut by God. But she cried to him and made a promise that if he would bless her womb with a son, that she would offer him back to him, that he may serve God all his life. A year later she returned to the Temple with a baby boy in her hand. And when he was 5 years old, she handed him over into the care of the priest as she had promised. Samuel grew up in the temple and became one of the greatest and most revered prophets of God who would lead Israel for 40 years. And when Hannah gave her only begotten son back to God for his service, Eli the High Priest blessed Elkanah and his wife, and said, The Lord give you the seed of this woman, for the loan which is lent to the Lord. And they went back to their home. And the Lord visited Hannah, so that she conceived, and bear three more sons and two daughters. And the child Samuel grew before the Lord.

Then there was another woman of great importance, yet her name was never mentioned. She had a spirit of hospitality and when she saw a stranger passing by, she invited him to stay over. Eventually, she perceived that this man was a holy man and after consulting with her husband she prepared him a room to rest there on his frequent travels. So, one day the prophet Elisha wanted to repay her in kindness, but she was content. His servant informed him that the woman had no child and that her husband was old. So, Elisha called her and said she would have a baby around the same time the following year. Shocked by what she heard, she responded, no, my lord, you are a man of God, do not lie to me. And it did come to pass according to the word of the prophet that she did bear a son.

So, no matter what your age or medical report. Whose report will you believe? Let not your heart despair because of an empty womb. Hear the word of the Lord, and only believe. He opens and closes the wombs as in the days of old. For with God, nothing shall be impossible. And as Elizabeth heard the greetings of Mary the baby in her womb leaped. And she spoke with a loud voice saying, blessed are you among women, and blessed is the fruit of your womb. And blessed is she who believes, for there will be a performance of those things which were told her, from the Lord. Hallelujah, my soul magnifies the Lord. May your womb, and your seed be blessed in Jesus' name. Amen.

14. COVID TERROR

Like inmates behind bars, so are my friends and I in lockdown. Freedoms clipped like bird's wings, isolated into familiar spaces, while some, lying in foreign beds, fighting death with every breath.

Bill Gates did a Corona Edtalk, but his hypothesis would not persuade casual men to prevent the Covid Terror. And WHO would not prepare for a pandemic until the Wuhan rumors turned deadly around the world. A perfect storm of fear and frenzy, forcing social distancing, six feet away or under by an invisible force. Yet some protested amendment rights, forgetting peace and love for one's neighbor is the greater commandment from above.

But though I walk through the valley of the shadow of death, I will fear no evil. Bloody Friday paraded death as a champion, but by Easter Sunday, Christ's resurrection power crushed his pride and his head. Followed by a worldwide tweet saying, Jesus is alive, believe this gospel, and be baptized.

15. THE HEALTHY BODY

I will take sickness away from you and heal you from all your wounds. No sickness or disease will cling to your body. Trust me for I have send my word to heal you. No need to cling to medication as your source of health. For my word is medicine to all your flesh. Only believe. Take my word for your daily dose of vitamins. Receive my instructions for your health. Believe my word. For I was wounded for your transgression, i was bruised for your iniquities, and by my stripes you are healed. No need to depend on tablets and prescription for your life does not depend on it. Many have died in perfect health and without my word their health and hope has vanished. No my word has not only promise for health in this life, but also eternal life even if you die in faith.

Your healthcare does not cover sin-sick souls. And reducing body fat is not the healthier solution to looking skinny good. A healthy mind and body make a happy soul, but a spirit void of virtue is as unhealthy as fat fast foods. If you are serious about finding a better-looking you, look no more. You have found the right channel where Botox is unnecessary, where you will be loved and accepted for what you were created to be. God's word works like medicine. Take it daily. In a twinkling of an eye, the corruptible will change into incorruptible, and the mortal will change into immortality. For what does it profit anyone to gain bodily perfection yet lose his or her soul? From the sole of their feet to the head there was nothing sound in it. Only bruises, welts, and raw wounds, not bandaged or softened with oil. But no matter how sick society has become, there is hope from God to heal. God's word is life to those who find them and health to all their flesh. As it is written, He that believes in me, as the scripture says, out of his belly shall flow rivers of living water.

1. HEALTHY HEADS

1. The Lord will make you the head and not the tail. Deuteronomy 28:13

2. You anoint my head with oil. Psalm 23:5

3. You kept me as head of the nations. 2 Samuel 22:44

4. His mischief will return upon his own head. And his violence will descend upon his own pate. Psalm 7:16

5. If your enemy is hungry feed him, and if he is thirsty give him a drink. For in so doing you will heap coals of fire on his head. Romans 12:20

6. The very hairs of your head are all numbered. Do not fear, for you are more valuable than many sparrows. Luke 12:7

7. Blessings are on the head of the just. Proverbs 10:6

8. The husband is the head of the wife, as Christ also is the head of the church. Ephesians 5:23

9. The Lord will bind up the breach of his people and heal the stroke of their wounds. Isaiah 30:26

10. It shall come to pass in that day that his burden will be taken away from your shoulder, and his yoke from your neck, and the yoke will be destroyed because of the anointing oil. Isaiah 10:27

11. He crowns me with loving kindness and tender mercies. Psalm 103:4

2. HEALTHY FACES

1. And the Lord spoke face to face with Moses as a man would speak to his friend. Numbers 12:8

2. My face is dirty with weeping, and my eyelids are like the shadow of death. Job 16:16

3. They looked to him and were lightened, and their faces were not ashamed. Psalm 34:5

4. A merry heart makes a cheerful face. Proverbs 15:13

5. And you with open face beholding as in a glass the glory of the Lord and is changed into the same image from glory to glory by the Spirit of the Lord. 2 Corinthians 3:18

6. The Lord God will help me, therefore shall I not be confounded. I have set my face like a flint, and I know that I shall not be ashamed. Isaiah 50:7

7. Be not afraid of their faces, for I am with you to deliver you, says the Lord. Jeremiah 1:8

8. Beauty is vain, and charm is deceitful, but a woman who fears the Lord will be praised. Proverbs 31:30

3. HEALTHY MINDS

1. Then he opened their understanding, that they might understand the scriptures. Luke 24:45

2. Who has known the mind of the Lord, that he may instruct him? But you have the mind of Christ. 1 Corinthians 2:16

3. Make me of quick understanding in the fear of the Lord. Isaiah 11:3

4. The memory of the just is blessed. Proverbs 10:7

5. My meditation of him will be sweet. Psalm 104:34

6. You keep him in perfect peace, whose mind is stayed on you because he trusts in you. Isaiah 26:3

7. And the peace of God that passes all understanding will keep your heart and mind through Christ Jesus. Finally, whatsoever things are true, honest, just, pure, lovely, and of a good report, and if there be any virtue or praise, think on these things. Philippians 4:8

8. Be not conformed to this world, but transform yourself by the renewing of your mind, and so prove what is the good, acceptable, and perfect will of God. Romans 12:2

9. Be renewed in the spirit of your mind. Ephesians 4:23-24

10. To be carnally minded is death, but to be spiritually minded is life and peace. Romans 8:6

11. The thoughts of the righteous are right. Proverbs 12:5

12. The thoughts of the diligent tend to plentiful. Proverbs 21:5

13. You have an unction from the Holy One and know all things. 1 John 2:19

14. The Holy Ghost teaches me and puts me in remembrance of all Jesus said. John 14.26

4. HEALTHY EYES

1. Hear you deaf and look you blind that you may see. Who is blind, like my servant? Or deaf as my messenger that I send? Who is blind as he that is perfect, and blind as the Lord's servant? Isaiah 42:18

2. The eyes of the wicked will fail. Job 11:20

3. The light of the eyes rejoices the heart. Proverbs 15:30

4. The eyes of Moses did not dim till his death. Deuteronomy 34:7

5. Then he touched their eyes, and said, let it be according to your faith. And their eyes were opened. Matthew 9:27

6. Lord, enlighten my eyes. Proverbs 29:13

7. The eyes of them that see will not be dim, and the ears of them that hear will hear. Isaiah 32:3

8. Be not wise in your own eyes but fear the Lord and depart from evil. Proverbs 3:6

9. Give me your heart and let your eyes observe my ways. Proverbs 23:26

10. My eyes have seen the King, the Lord of hosts. Isaiah 6:5

11. Eyes have not seen, and ears have not heard, nor has entered into the heart of man the things which God has prepared for those who love him. 1 Corinthians 2:9

12. Since the world began was it not heard that any man opened the eyes of one that was born blind. But a man called Jesus made clay and anointed my eyes and said to me, Go to the pool of Siloam and wash. So I went and washed, and I received my sight. John 9

13. See how my eyes have been enlightened when I tasted a little of

this honey. 1 Samuel 14:25

14. And Jesus asked him, what do you want me to do for you? And the blind man said, Teacher, I want to see. And Jesus said to him, Go your way, your faith has made you well. And immediately he received his sight. Mark 10:46

15. Stand and see this great thing, which the Lord will do before your eyes. 1 Samuel 12:16

16. Blessed are your eyes for they see, and your ears for they hear. Matthew 13:6

17. And they brought a blind man to him and begged him to touch him. He then took the hand of the blind man and led him out of the town. And having spit on his eyes and putting his hands on him, he asked him if he saw anything. And the man looked up and said, I see men like trees walking around. Again he placed his hands on his eyes and made him look up. And he was restored and saw everyone clearly. Mark 8:22

18. The commandment of the Lord is pure, enlightening the eyes. Psalm 19:8

19. Keep my commandments and live, and my teachings as the apple of your eye. Proverbs 7:2

20. I counsel you, buy from me gold tried in the fire that you may be rich, and white robes that you may be clothed that the shame of your nakedness do not appear, and anoint your eyes with eye salve that you may see. Revelation 3:18

21. Then the eyes of the blind shall be opened, and the ears of the deaf unstopped. Isaiah 35:5

22. I am the Lord, I have called you in righteousness. I will take you by the hand and keep you, I will give you as a covenant for the people, a light for the nations, to open the eyes that are blind, to bring out the prisoners from the dungeon, and from prison those who sit in darkness. Isaiah 42:6

23. Out of their gloom and darkness the eyes of the blind will

see. Isaiah 29:18

24. And I will lead the blind in a way that they do not know and in paths that they have not known. I will guide them. I will turn darkness before them into light, the rough places I will level to the ground. These are the things I do, and I do not forsake them. Isaiah 42:16

25. The Lord opens the eyes of the blind. Psalm 146:8

26. Jesus said, For judgment I came into this world that those who do not see may see, and those who see may become blind. John 9:39

27. And the blind and the lame came to him in the temple, and he healed them. Matthew 21:14

28. And two blind men followed him, crying aloud, Have mercy on us, Son of David. And when he entered the house, the blind men came to him, and Jesus said to them, Do you believe that I can to do this? They said to him, Yes Lord. Then he touched their eyes, saying, According to your faith be it done unto you. And their eyes were opened. Matthew 9:27

29. And a demon-oppressed man, who was blind and mute, was brought to him, and he healed him so that the man spoke and saw. Matthew 12:22

30. The Spirit of the Lord is upon me because he has anointed me to proclaim good news to the poor. He has sent me to proclaim liberty to the captives and recovering of sight to the blind, to set at liberty those who are oppressed. Luke 4:18

31. Then will the eyes of those who see, not be closed, and the ears of those who hear give attention. Isaiah 32:3

32. Why do you behold the mote in your brother's eyes, but do not see the beam in your own eyes? Luke 6:41

33. He that has a bountiful eye shall be blessed. Proverbs 22:9

34. And their eyes were opened, and they knew him, and he vanished out of their sight. Luke 24:31

35. You will see the glory of God. John 11:18

36. My eyes have seen your salvation. Luke 2:30

37. Your eyes will see the king in his beauty. Isaiah 33:17

38. I will set no wicked thing before mine eyes. Psalm 101:3

39. I made a covenant with my eyes. Job 31:1

40. And immediately there fell something like scales from his eyes and he received sight, and he rose and was baptized. Acts 9:18

41. I speak to them in parables though seeing they see not, and hearing they hear not, neither do they understand. Matthew 13:13

42. The light of the body is the eye: if therefore thine eye be single, thy whole body shall be full of light. Matthew 6:22

43. The Lord opens the eyes of the blind. Psalm 146:8

44. And in that day shall the deaf hear the words of the book, and the eyes of the blind shall see out of obscurity, and out of darkness. Isaiah 29:18

45. And he put his hands again upon his eyes, and made him look up and he was restored, and saw every man clearly. Mark 8:25

46. Then the eyes of the blind shall be opened, and the ears of the deaf shall be unstopped. Isaiah 35:5

47. The hearing ear, and the seeing eye, the Lord hath made even both of them. Proverbs 20:12

48. Open my eyes, that I may behold wondrous things out of your law. Psalm 119:18

49. I send you to open their eyes and to turn them from darkness to light, and from the power of Satan unto God, that they may receive forgiveness of sins, and an inheritance among them which are sanctified by faith that is in Me. Acts 26:18

50. May the God of our Lord Jesus Christ, the Father of glory, give unto you the spirit of wisdom and revelation in the knowledge of him, the eyes of your understanding being enlightened that you may know what is the hope of his calling, and what the riches of the glory of his inheritance in the saints. Ephesians 1:17-18

51. And Elisha prayed, and said, Lord, I pray you, open his eyes, that he may see. And the Lord opened the eyes of the young man and he saw. And, behold, the mountain was full of horses and chariots of fire round about Elisha. And when they came down to him, Elisha prayed unto the Lord, and said, Smite this people, I pray with blindness. And he smote them with blindness according to the word of Elisha. And Elisha said unto them, This is not the way, neither is this the city. Follow me, and I will bring you to the man whom you seek. But he led them to Samaria. And it came to pass, when they came into Samaria, that Elisha said, Lord, open the eyes of these men, that they may see. And the Lord opened their eyes, and they saw that they were in the midst of Samaria. 2 Kings 6:17-20

5. HEALTHY MOUTHS

1. Be not rash with your mouth, and let not your heart be hasty to utter anything before God. For God is in heaven, and you are upon the earth. Therefore, let your words be few and suffer not your mouth to cause your flesh to sin. Neither say to the angel, it was an error. Why should God be angry at your voice, and destroy the work of your hands? Ecclesiastes 5:2

2. The Lord God has given me the tongue of the learned, that I should know how to speak a word in season to him that is weary. Isaiah 50:4

3. You satisfy my mouth with good things. Psalm 103:5

4. Immediately his mouth was opened and his tongue loosed, and he spoke, praising God. Luke 1:64

5. She opens her mouth with wisdom and on her tongue is the law of kindness. Proverbs 31:26

6. The mouth of the righteous speaks wisdom and his tongue talk of judgment. Psalm 37:30

7. My mouth will speak wisdom. Psalm 49:3

8. The words of his mouth were smoother than butter, but war was in his heart. His words were softer than oil, yet were they like drawn swords. Psalm 55:21

9. The things that go out of the mouth come forth from the heart, and that defiles the man. Matthew 15:18

10. He will make you a new sharp threshing instrument having teeth. Isaiah 41:15

11. He makes my mouth like a sharp sword. Isaiah 49:2

12. Out of the abundance of the heart the mouth speaks. Luke 6:45

13. Everything that has breath, praise the Lord. Psalm 150:6

14. Woe is me! for I am a man of unclean lips, and I dwell among people with unclean lips. Isaiah 6:5

15. My lips will not speak wickedness, nor will my tongue utter deceit. Job 27:4

16. My lips greatly rejoice as I sing to you. Psalm 71:23

17. These people draw close to me with their mouths and honor me with their lips, but their hearts are far from me. Matthew 15:8

18. Let the words of my mouth and the meditation of my heart be acceptable in your sight, o Lord my strength, and my redeemer. Psalm 19:14

19. Put away from you a froward mouth and perverse lips. Proverbs 4:24

20. The tongue of the stammerers will speak plainly. Isaiah 32:4

21. Open your mouth and I will fill it. Psalm 81:10

22. Fill my mouth with laughter and my lips with rejoicing. Job 8:21

23. My mouth will declare your righteousness and salvation. Psalm 71:15

24. My words are from the uprightness of my heart that my lips may utter knowledge clearly. Job 33:3

25. Life and death is in the power of my tongue. Proverbs 18:21

26. My lips utter praise when you teach me your statutes. My tongue speak your word for all your commandments are righteousness. Psalm 119:171

27. I create the fruit of the lips. says the Lord Isaiah 57:18

28. My mouth will speak to praise the Lord. Psalm 145:21

29. Love not in words and tongue, but in deed and in truth. 1 John 3:18

30. The tongue no man can tame, it is unruly, evil, and full of poison. Out of the same mouth, you bless God and curse men. This

should not be. James 3: 5

31. The lips of knowledge are a beautiful jewel. Proverbs 20:15

32. Then the Lord put forth his hand and touched my mouth. And the Lord said unto me, Behold, I have put my words in thy mouth. Jeremiah 1:9

33. I will give you a mouth and wisdom which all your adversaries shall not be able to refute nor resist. Luke 21:15

34. I have put my words in your mouth, and I have covered you in the shadow of my hand. Isaiah 59:16

35. So will be the word that goes out of my mouth. It shall not return unto me void but shall accomplish that which I please and shall prosper in the things to whereto I sent it. Isaiah 55:11

36. My spirit is on you, and my words which I have put in your mouth will not depart out of your mouth, nor out of the mouth of your seed, nor out of the mouth of your seed's seed, says the Lord, from now until forever. Isaiah 59:21

37. I will speak of excellent things and the opening of my lips shall be right things. My mouth shall speak truth and wickedness is an abomination to my lips. All the words of my mouth are in righteousness and there is nothing froward or perverse in them. Proverbs 8:6

38. I have preached righteousness in the great congregation. I have not refrained my lips. Lord, you know. Psalm 40:9

39. A man is satisfied with good by the fruit of his mouth. Proverbs 12:14

40. How sweet are your words to my taste, yeah, sweeter than honey to my mouth. Psalm 119:103

41. The tongue of the wise is health. Proverbs 13:18

42. He has put a new song in my mouth to praise God. Many will see it, and fear, and will trust in the Lord. Psalm 40:3

43. My lips will greatly rejoice when I sing to you, and my soul which you have redeemed. My tongue also will speak of your

righteousness all day long. Psalm 71:23

6. HEALTHY EARS

1. Let every man be swift to hear, slow to speak, and slow to wrath. James 1:19

2. The hearing ear and the seeing eye, the Lord made them both. Proverbs 20:12

3. He that has an ear, let him hear what the Spirit says to the church. Revelation 2:7

4. But they refused to listen and pulled away their shoulders, and stopped their ears, that they should not hear. Zechariah 7:11

5. Then he said to them, this day is this scripture fulfilled in your ears. Luke 4:21

6. He that planted the ear, will he not hear? And he who formed the eye, shall he not see? Psalm 94:9

7. I have heard of you by the hearing of the ear, but now my eyes have seen you. Job 42:5

8. He awakens me morning by morning, he awakens my ear to hear as the learned. He opened my ear, and I was not rebellious nor turned my back. Isaiah 50:4

9. In that day the deaf shall hear the words of a book. Isaiah 29:18

10. But I, as a deaf man, heard not. I was like a dumb man that opened not his mouth. Psalm 38:13

11. And they brought unto him one that was deaf and had an impediment in his speech. And they beseech him to put his hand upon him. And he took him aside from the multitude, and put his fingers into his ears, and he spit, and touched his tongue. And looking up to heaven, he sighed, and said to him, Ephphatha,

that is, Be opened. And straightway his ears were opened, and the string of his tongue was loosed, and he spake plain. Mark 7: 32

12. My ears you have opened. Psalm 40:6

13. He that has an ear, let him hear. Mark 7:16

7. HEALTHY HANDS

1. I the Lord God will hold your right hand, saying, fear not, I will help you. Isaiah 41:13

2. If iniquity is in your hand, put it far away. Job 11:14

3. He will deliver the islands of the innocent, for it is delivered by the pureness of their hands. Job 22:30

4. Lift up your hands in the sanctuary and bless the Lord. Psalm 134:2

5. Let the beauty of the Lord God be upon you and establish the work of your hands. Psalm 90:17

6. He that has clean hands will be stronger and stronger. Job 17:9

7. He teaches my hands to war so that a bow of steel is broken by mine arms. 2 Samuel 22:35

8. The hand of the diligent shall bear rule. Proverbs 12:24

9. And the hand of the diligent makes rich. Proverbs 10:4

10. Be strong and let not your hands be weak, for your work will be rewarded. 2 Chronicles 15:7

11. The recompense of a man's hand shall in return return to him. Proverb 12:14

12. He laid his hands on every one of them and healed them. Luke 4:40

13. Now He could do no mighty work there, except that He laid His hands on a few sick people and healed them. Mark 6:5

14. You will lay hands on the sick, and they will recover. Mark 16:18

8. HEALTHY FEET

1. Simon Peter said to Jesus, Lord, then wash not only my feet but my hands and my head also. John 13:9

2. Her feet go down to death and her steps will take you to hell. Proverbs 5:5

3. How beautiful are the feet of them who bring good news. Isaiah 52:7

4. Turn not to the right or left but remove your foot from evil. Proverbs 4:24

5. How beautiful are your feet with shoes, my princess daughter? The joints of your thighs are like jewels, the work of the hands of a cunning workman. Songs of Solomon 7:1

6. Your word is a lamp to my feet and a light to my path. Psalm 119:105

7. My feet will stand in your gates, O Jerusalem. Psalm 122:2

8. But the father said to his servants, Bring forth the best robe, and put it on him and put a ring on his hand, and shoes on his feet. Luke 15:22

9. HEALTHY BONES

1. And Elisha the prophet died and was buried. And it came to pass while burying another man, that they spotted the enemy and decided to abandon his body in the grave of Elisha. And when the corps that was let down touched Elisha's bones, he revived and stood up on his feet. 2 Kings 13:20

2. When I kept silent my bones waxed old, and because your hand was heavy upon me, my moisture turned into the drought of summer. Psalm 32:3-4

3. There is no soundness in my flesh because of your anger, and no rest in my bones because of my sin. Psalm 38:3

4. A good report makes the bones fat. Proverbs 15:30

5. A merry heart does good like medicine, but a broken spirit dries the bones. Proverbs 17:22

6. He keeps all my bones, not one of them is broken. Psalm 34:20

7. Make me to hear joy and gladness, that the bones which you have broken may rejoice. Psalm 51:8

8. And Job sinned not with his lips when Satan smote his bones and flesh with sore boils. Job 2:4-10

9. A happy heart works like medicine, but a broken spirit dries up the bones. Proverbs 17:22

10. His word was in my heart as a burning fire shut up in my bones. Jeremiah 20:9

11. Fear the Lord, and depart from evil. It will be health to thy navel and marrow to thy bones. Proverbs 3:7,8

12. The light of the eyes rejoices the heart, and a good report

makes the bones fat. Proverbs 15:30

13. Envy rotten the bones. Proverbs 14:30

14. The hand of the Lord was upon me, and carried me out in the spirit of the Lord, and set me down in the midst of the valley which was full of bones. And he caused me to pass by them roundabout, and behold, there were many in the open valley and they were very dry. And he said to me, Son of man, can these bones live? And I answered, O Lord God, thou know. Then he said to me, Prophesy over these bones, and say to them, Dry bones, hear the word of the Lord. Thus says the Lord God to these bones. I will cause breath to enter into you, and you shall live. And I will lay sinews upon you, and will bring up flesh upon you, and cover you with skin, and put breath in you, and you will live, and you will know that I am the Lord.

So I prophesied as I was commanded. And as I prophesied, there was a noise and a shaking, and the bones came together, bone to his bone. And I beheld, sinews and flesh came upon them, and skin covered them, but there was no breath in them. Then he said to me, Prophesy to the wind, son of man, and say to the wind, Thus saith the Lord God, Come from the four winds, O breath, and breathe upon these slain, that they may live. So I prophesied as he commanded, and breath came into them and they lived, and stood up upon their feet, an exceeding great army. Then he said unto me, Son of man, these bones are the whole house of Israel. Behold, they say, Our bones are dry and our hope is lost. We are cut off for our part. But prophesy and say to them, Thus saith the Lord God: My people, I will open your graves, and cause you to come up out of your graves, and bring you into the land of Israel. And you shall know that I am the Lord, when I have opened your graves my people, and have brought you up out of your graves. And I will put my spirit in you, and you shall live, and I shall place you in your own land, then shall you know that I the Lord have spoken it, and performed it, says the Lord. Ezekiel 37:1-14

10. HEALTHY HEARTS

1. My child, forget not my law, but let your heart keep my commandments. Trust in the Lord with all your heart and lean not unto your own understanding. Proverbs 3:1-5

2. Keep your heart with all diligence, for out of it flows the issues of life. Proverbs 4:21-23

3. I will walk within my house with a perfect heart. Psalm 101:2

4. With a perfect heart the people offered willingly to the Lord. 1 Chronicles 29:9

5. The heart that seeks God will live. Psalm 69:32

6. God, make my heart soft. Job 23:16

7. I found a man after my own heart. Acts 13:22

8. Create in me a clean heart oh God, and renew in me a right spirit. Psalm 51:10

9. Let your heart retain my words. Keep my commandments and live. Proverbs 4:4

10. I will give you a new heart. Ezekiel 36:26

11. Let not your heart be troubled. You believe in God, believe also in me. John 14:1

12. The heart of the rash will understand knowledge. Isaiah 32:3

13. Hope deferred makes the heart sick, but when the desire comes it is a tree of life. Proverbs 13:12

14. Be of good courage and he will strengthen your heart. Psalm 31:24

15. A man's heart devises his way, but the Lord directs his steps. Proverbs 16:9

16. The Lord searches the heart. Jeremiah 17:10

17. God knows the secrets of the heart. Psalm 44:21

18. My heart is broken. Jeremiah 23:9

19. A sound heart is the life of the flesh. Proverbs 14:30

20. My heart trembles and is moved out of its place. Job 37:1

21. A broken and contrite heart, o God you will not despise. Psalm 50:17

22. He heals the brokenhearted and binds up their wounds. Psalm 51:17

23. He sent me to heal the brokenhearted. Luke 4:18

24. Good words makes glad the heart. Proverbs 12:25

25. In the uprightness of my heart I did this. 1 Chronicles 29:17

26. Delight yourself in the Lord and he will give you the desires of your heart. Psalm 37:4

27. Apply your heart to understanding. Proverbs 2:2

28. I will give them a heart to know Me, and they will return to Me, with all their heart. Jeremiah 24:7

29. Your heart is where your treasure is. Matthew 6:21

30. God knowing their hearts, purified their hearts by faith. Acts 15:9

31. Love one another with a pure heart. 1 Peter 1:22

32. Blessed are the pure in heart for they will see God. Matthew 5:8

33. Lord you know me, and see me, and test my heart toward you. Jeremiah 12:3

34. You know the hearts of everyone. 1 Kings 8:39

35. Remove their hearts of stone and give them hearts of flesh. Ezekiel 36:26

36. I will write My law in their heart. Hebrews 10:16

37. Let not your heart be troubled nor be afraid. John 14:27

38. Establish my heart unblameable in holiness. 1 Thessalonians 3:13

10. HEALTHY HEARTS

39. If your heart condemns you God is greater than your heart. And if your heart condemns you not, then you will have confidence with God. 1 John 3:20

40. A good man out of the good treasure of his heart brings forth good and an evil man out of the evil treasure of his heart brings forth evil. And out of the abundance of the heart the mouth speaks. Luke 6:45

41. My heart trusts in him, and I am helped. Therefore my heart greatly rejoices and with songs will I praise him. Psalm 28:7

42. It was in your heart to build a house for my name, and you did well that it was in your heart. 1 Kings 8:18

43. Let your heart be perfect with the Lord your God, to walk in his statutes, and to keep his commandments. 1 Kings 8:61

44. The Lord sees not as man sees. For man looks on the outside appearance, but the Lord looks at the heart. 1 Samuel 16:7

45. But you have obeyed from the heart that form of doctrine which was delivered to you. Romans 6:17

46. The law of God is in his heart, none of his steps will slide. Psalm 37:31

47. And they said one to another, did not our hearts burn within us, when he talked with us on the way while he opened to us the scriptures? Luke 24:32

48. My heart trust in him and I am helped. Therefore my heart greatly rejoice, and with song will I praise him. Psalm 28:7

49. I delight to do your will my God, for your law is within my heart. Psalm 40:8

50. Fear not, from the first day that you set your heart to understand and chasten yourself before God, your words were heard, and I came because of your words. Daniel 10:12

51. God knows the heart of every man. Acts 1:24

52. Wine makes glad the heart. Psalm 104:15

53. Sorrow is better than laughter for by the sadness of the countenance the heart is made better. The heart of the wise is in the house of mourning, but the heart of fools is in the house of mirth. Ecclesiastes 7:3-4

54. Know the God of your father, and serve him with a perfect heart and with a willing mind. For the Lord searches all hearts and understands all the imaginations of the thoughts. If you seek him, you will find him but if you forsake him, he will cast you off for ever. 1 Chronicles 28:9

55. Believe with your heart that God raised Jesus from the dead and you will be saved. For with the heart, man believes unto righteousness and with his mouth, he confesses unto salvation. Romans 10: 9-10

11. HEALTHY AGE

1. The Lord has kept me alive, as he said. It is 45 years since the Lord spoke this word to Moses. Today I am 85 years old, and I am still as strong this day as I was on the day that Moses sent me. As my strength was then, even so, is my strength now for war, both to go out, and to come in again. Joshua 14:10

2. You are my trust, from my youth. Psalm 71:5

3. Moses was 120 years old when he died. His eyes did not dim, nor did his natural force abate. Deuteronomy 34:7

4. He died a good old age, full of days, riches, and honor. 1 Chronicles 29:28

5. Your age will be clearer than the noonday. You will shine forth like the morning. Job 11:17

6. To your old age I am he, even to your grey hairs will I carry you and will deliver you. Isaiah 46:4

7. You will come to your grave at a full age. Job 5:26

8. You will still bring forth fruit in your old age and will be fat and flourishing. Psalm 92:14

9. He renews your youth like that of an eagle. Psalm 103:5

10. You have made my days as a hand breadth, and my age is as nothing before you. Every man at his best state is altogether vanity. Psalm 39:5

11. I have been young and now am old, yet have I not seen the righteous forsaken nor his seed begging bread. Psalm 37:25

12. And Sarah was 127 years old when she died after she had the promised child at age 99. Genesis 23:1

13. And the years of Abraham's life that he lived was 175 years. Then Abraham gave up the ghost, and died in a good old age, an old man, and full of years and was gathered to his people. Genesis 25:7

14. After this Job lived 140 years and saw his sons and his grandchildren up to the fourth generation. And Job died, being old, and full of days. Job 42:16

15. And all the days of Methuselah were 969 years, and he died. Genesis 5:27

16. And Enoch walked with God, and he was not, for God took him. Genesis 5:24

17. But if the Spirit of him that raised up Jesus from the dead dwell in you, he that raised up Christ from the dead shall also quicken your mortal bodies by his Spirit that dwell in you. Romans 8:11

18. When I am old and grey-headed God, forsake me not until I have shown your strength to this generation and your power to everyone that is to come. Psalm 71:18

19. Walk in my ways, and I will lengthen your days. 1 Kings 3:14

12. HEALTHY BABIES

1. Moses and Jesus were both born at a time when kings ordered the slaughter of babies. Both men were supernaturally protected by God to become the greatest lawgivers in human history. Exodus and Matthew

2. The Lord has called me from the womb. From the bowels of my mother, he made mention of my name. Isaiah 49:1

3. The Lord will give you a sign. A virgin will conceive and bear a son and call his name Emmanuel. Isaiah 7:14

4. And the virgin Mary was found with child of the Holy Spirit and gave birth to the savior of the world. Matthew 1:18-25

5. The Lord has closed the womb of Hannah, but after her prayer and bitter tears, the Lord remembered her and gave her a son, called Samuel, who became one of Israel's greatest prophets. 1 Samuel 1

6. Cursed be the day I was born, cursed be the man who brought the good news to my father because he slew me not in the womb of my mother, that her body would have been my grave. Jeremiah 20:14-18

7. And the midwives feared God and did not kill the babies as the king of Egypt commanded. Exodus 1: 17-22

8. In the beginning God made man in his own likeness and image. And Adam knew his wife Eve who gave birth in pain because of the curse. Genesis 3

9. And he will be filled with the Holy Ghost in his mother's womb. Luke 1:15

10. Thus says the Lord, I have healed the waters. There shall be no more any death or barren land. 2 Kings 2:21

11. So Abraham prayed to God, and God healed Abimelech, his wife, and his maidservants, and they bore children. Genesis 20:17

12. Abram was childless because Sarai his wife bore him no children. Then the Lord visited Sarah as he had said, and did as he has spoken. Genesis 21:1

13. Through faith Sarah herself received strength to conceive seed and delivered a child when she was past age. Hebrews 11:11

14. Before I formed you in the belly I knew you, and before you came out of the womb I sanctified you, and ordained you as a prophet to the nations. Jeremiah 1:5

13. HEALTHY SOULS AND SPIRITS

1. My servant Caleb has another spirit in him and followed me fully. Him will I bring into the land and his seed shall possess it. Numbers 24:14

2. The Lord lives who has made the soul. Jeremiah 38:16

3. He that is joined to the Lord is one spirit. 1 Corinthians 6:17

4. You have not received the spirit of bondage again to fear, but you have received the Spirit of adoption that cries out Abba Father. Romans 8:15

5. God fills the weary soul and replenishes every sorrowful soul. Jeremiah 31:25

6. A man's spirit sustains him in his infirmity, but a wounded spirit who can bear. Proverbs 18:14

7. Be not hasty in spirit to be angry, for anger sits in the bosom of fools. Ecclesiastes 7:9

8. This is vanity and a vexation of the spirit. Ecclesiastes 6:9

9. Beloved, I wish above all things that you may prosper and be in health, even as your soul prospers. 3 John 2

10. May the God of our Lord Jesus Christ, the Father of glory, give you a spirit of wisdom and of revelation in the knowledge of him. Ephesians 1:17

11. If the Spirit of of him who raised Jesus from the dead dwells in you, He who raised Christ from the dead, will also quicken your mortal body by His Spirit that dwells in you. Romans 8:11

12. You have delivered my soul from death, my eyes from tears, and my feet from falling. Psalm 116:8

13. I receive beauty for ashes, the oil of joy for mourning, and I put on the garment of praise for the spirit of heaviness. Isaiah 61:3

14. And she was in bitterness of soul and prayed unto the Lord and wept sore. 1 Samuel 1:10

15. Bless the Lord oh my soul and all that is within me bless his holy name. Psalm 103:1

16. I am full of a matter, but the spirit within me constrains me. Job 33:18

17. For the word of God is quick and powerful, and sharper than a two-edged sword, piercing even to the dividing asunder of the soul and spirit, and of the joints and marrow, and is a discerner of the thoughts and intends of the heart. Hebrews 4:12

18. And the Lord God formed man of the dust of the ground and breathed into his nostrils the breath of life. And man became a living soul. Genesis 2:7

19. It's the Spirit that quickens, but the flesh profits nothing. The words that I speak to you are spirit and life. John 6:63

20. He that gets wisdom loves his own soul. Proverbs 19:8

21. Let not your soul spare for his crying. Proverbs 19:18

22. The spirit of a man is the candle of the Lord who searches the inward parts of the belly. Proverbs 20:27

23. The blueness of a wound cleanses away evil and so do stripes in the inward parts of the belly. Proverbs 20:30

24. For you are bought with a price. Therefore glorify God in your body, and in your spirit, which are God's. 1 Corinthians 6:20

25. Into your hand I commit my spirit. Psalm 31:5

14. GOD'S BODY

1. God created man in **his image**, and in **his likeness** God created them. Genesis 1:27

2. In the beginning was the Word, and the Word was with God, and the Word was God. And the Word was made **flesh** and dwelt among us. John 1:14

2. His **eyes** are upon the ways of man, and he sees all his doings. Job 34:21

3. He endured, as **seeing Him** who is unseen. Hebrews 11:27

4. I have seen the angel of the Lord **face to face**. Judges 6:22

5. Manoah said to his wife, we will surely die, for **we have seen God**. Judges 13:22

6. Pity me for **the hand of God** touched me. Job 19:21

7. Remove your stroke away from me. For I am consumed by **the blow of your hand**. Psalm 39:10

8. The **eyes of the Lord** are on them that fear him. Psalm 33:18

9. The **fourth person** with them in the furnace is like the Son of God. Daniel 3:25

10. He put all things in subjection **under his feet** and gave him to be **the head** over all things to the church. Ephesians 1:22

11. **Christ is the head** of man and **God is the head** of Christ. 1 Corinthians 11:3

12. By **the word of the Lord** were the heavens made, and all the host by **the breath of his mouth**. Psalm 33:6

13. The magicians said to Pharaoh, this is **the finger of God**. Exodus 8:19

14. I saw **the Lord sitting** upon his throne, high and lifted up and his train filled the temple. Isaiah 6:1

15. **The eyes of the Lord** are upon the righteous, and **his ears** are open to their cry. But **the face of the Lord** is against them that do evil. Psalm 34:15

16. Hide me in **the secret of your presence.** Psalm 31:20

17. Behold, the name of the Lord comes from afar burning with his anger, and its burden is heavy. **His lips** are full of indignation, and **his tongue** as a devouring fire. And **his breath**, as an overflowing stream. Isaiah 30:27

18. The Lord gives wisdom. Out of **his mouth** comes knowledge and understanding. Proverbs 3:6

19. I will be glorious in **the eyes** of the Lord. Isaiah 49:5

20. I have graven you on **the palm of my hands.** Isaiah 49:16

21. I will perform the intents of **my heart.** Jeremiah 30:24

22. My sheep hear **my voice** and they follow me. And I give to them eternal life and they will never perish, neither will any man pluck them out of **my hand**. My Father gave them to me and is greater than all. No man is able to pluck them out of **my Father's hands.** John 10:27

23. He will not judge after **the sight of his eyes**, nor reprove after the hearing of **his ears.** Isaiah 11:3

24. With him **I speak** mouth to mouth plainly and not in dark speeches. And he saw **the Lord's silhouette.** Numbers 12:8

25. Keep me as the apple of your eye. He who touches you touches **the apple of his eye.** Zechariah 8:2

26. The Lord gave to me two tables of stones written with **the finger of God** and on them was written all the words, which the LORD spake. Deuteronomy 9:10

27. You have neither heard **his voice** at any time nor seen his shape. John 5:37

28. He who has seen me, has **seen the Father** also. John 14:9

29. I know the thoughts **I think** towards you, thoughts of peace and not for evil, to give you hope and a future. Jeremiah 29:11

30. He will smite the earth with the rod of **his mouth** and with the **breath of his lips** will he slay the wicked. Isaiah 11:4

31. My **eyes** and my **heart** will be there perpetually. 1 Kings 9:3

32. His **head and hair** are white like snow, **his eyes** like fire, **his feet** like brass as if burned in a furnace, **his voice** like many waters, and **his countenance** as the sun shining in its full strength. Revelations 1:13

33. Take my yoke upon you, and learn of me for I am meek and **lowly in heart** and you shall find rest for your soul. Matthew 11:29

34. The **voice of the Lord** is powerful. Psalm 29

35. And he was transfigured before them and **his face** shined as the sun, and his raiment was white as the light. Matthew 17:2

36. Make your **face** to shine on your servant. Psalm 119:135

37. The **eyes of the Lord** run to and fro throughout the whole earth to show himself strong on behalf of them whose heart is perfect towards him. 2 Chronicles 16:9

38. You have **pure eyes**. Habakkuk 1:13

39. The **eyes of the Lord** preserve knowledge. Proverbs 22:12

15. BODY PRAYER

Abba Father, thank you for anointing my **head** with fresh oil today. Thank you for blessing the work of my **hands**, and to lay them on the sick to be healed. Thank you for beautiful **feet** that bring the gospel of peace wherever you sent me. Thank you for opening my **eyes** to see your glory that fills the whole earth. Thank you for **ears** to hear what the Spirit of the Lord is saying to the church. Thank you for filling my **mouth** with good things, sharpening my **teeth**, and for beautifying my **lips** with kindness. Thank you for blessing my **tongue** to speak as the oracles of God, and not to curse what you have blessed. Thank you for a perfect **heart** to love and obey you, and for the **mind** of Christ to know your will. Thank you that you bless the **womb** and the **seed** of the righteous. Make them fruitful with joy in your kingdom. I praise and worship you in **Spirit** and in truth. Thank you that I am **a member** of the **body** of Christ, of which Jesus is the **head** of the church. I bless you Father in the name of Jesus Christ, Lord of all, and Ruler over all the nations, amen.

16. HEALTHY FOODS

He rained down manna on them to eat and gave them the corn of heaven. And men ate angels food when He sent them food to the full. Psalm 78:24-25

Food for Champions:

You are what you eat they say. If you want to live forever, you need to eat like a champion. Certain foods have superior nutritional value than general brands. But food alone will not sustain a man in the day of sickness or adversary. You may have a strong body or mental disposition, but people need more than food to sustain them on their deathbeds. That is why God says that his word is medicine to all your flesh. God's word is food that gives life and health to both your body and your soul. And whoever overcomes is invited to come and eat of the tree of life, which is in the midst of the paradise of God. Revelation 2:7

Food to Avoid:

The only food commands the apostles gave to the church was not to eat food that still has its blood in it, for life is in the blood, and eat not food offered to idols, for your conscience's sake.

Food for Love:

If what you eat is going to offend your weak faithed brother, then for love's sake do not eat that in front of him. And so, fulfill God's commandment. Some are free to drink wine, while Nazarene's prefer juice. Paul even advised Timothy to have a little wine for his constant tummy aches. You are free but let not your freedom cause a stumbling block to your brother.

Food that Kills:

Now the serpent was more subtle than any animal of the field which the Lord God made. And he said to the woman, Did God really say, you may not eat of all the trees that are in the garden? But she responded to the serpent, We may eat of all the fruit of the trees of the garden, except the fruit of the tree in the middle of the garden. Because God said, you will not eat of it, neither touch it, lest you die. And the serpent said to the woman, truly you will not die, die! God knows that on the day you eat of it, your eyes will be opened, and you will be as gods knowing good and evil. And when the woman saw that the tree was good for food and that it was pleasant to the eyes, a tree to be desired to make one wise, she took of the fruit thereof and ate, and gave also to her husband which was with her, and he did eat. And the eyes of both of them were opened, and they knew that they were naked.

Food for Thought:

Jesus said man will not live by bread alone but by every word that comes from the mouth of God. The same night in which the Lord Jesus was betrayed he took bread and when he had given thanks, he broke it and said: Take and eat for this is my body, which is broken for you. Do this in remembrance of me. In the same manner, he also took the cup, and supped, saying, this cup is the New Testament in my blood. Do this as often as you drink it, in remembrance of me. Your words I found and I ate them and your word was to me, joy and the rejoicing of my heart. For I am called by your name.

Food Approved:

Eat honey, my son, for it is good for you. Simple advice. No secondhand opinions or approval is necessary from the WHO or FDA. There is a lot of advice on what and what not to eat. Friends, family, and experts will tell you their opinions, and what they have learned. But the New Testament approves all food for eating when done in faith. Peter had a vision from the Lord to eat food considered unclean. Jews would never eat that. It's forbidden, he replied. But Jesus responded: Peter, do not call unclean what I made clean, eat! All food is good and to be eaten. When you receive it with thanksgiving and prayer, it is sanctified by his word. All food is sanctified by prayer. People who live to be 100 years or more do not eat according to today's forced nutrition. And the bible neither promotes good health through a vegetarian diet. Daniel abstained from the king's meat not because he was vegetarian, but because of his devotion to the Lord God. Proverbs says: Wisdom will increase your life and the fear of the Lord is the beginning of wisdom.

Food of Thanksgiving:

Take no thought for your life, what you will eat, or what you will drink. Nor for your body, what you will put on. Is not life more than food, and the body more than clothes? God knows you need these things. Serve the Lord God, and he will bless your bread, and your water and take sickness away from you. Father, thank you that you bless my food and drink, and for taking away sickness from me, in Jesus' name, Amen. Exodus 23:25

17. A PERFECT HEART

I went to see the doctor after I felt pain in my chest. Tests were made to determine the cause. And when the results came back, the doctor said to me: Your heart is perfect. I instantly knew her words were from God. When God tested David's heart, he concluded, This is a man after my own heart. The Bible often mentions people whose hearts were perfect. God searches the heart and tries the reins, to give to every man according to his ways and according to the fruit of his doings. What will your health report say after a visit to the Great Physician? In Jeremiah seventeen God deals with the heart of man. His overall conclusion is the heart of man is deceitful above all things and desperately wicked. Who can know it? David cried, Lord, create in me a clean heart, and renew in me a right spirit. The wrong spirit entered ten spies that prevented Israel from going into the promised land. They ended up dead in the desert never enjoying their inheritance. A wrong spirit towards people or God can clog the arteries of your heart. You will end up losing your passion for his presence and his house. Life's pleasures and things also clog the pathways for the Word and the Spirit to flow richly. He is a Physician and an expert on heart matters. If you have a problem, you can have a heart-to-heart talk with God. Let his counsel soften your heart. He will perform a heart transplant and take out the heart of stone and give you a heart of flesh. That you too can rejoice and with a perfect heart willingly offer to the Lord offerings and praise. It is time to draw near to God with a perfect heart, that your joy may be full. Diligently protect your heart for out of it flows the issues of life. God is love and love is the commandment that keeps a heart healthy.

18. HEART PROBLEMS

1. Circumcise your uncircumcised heart. Romans 2:29

2. The imaginations of man's heart are evil from his youth. Genesis 8:21

3. They tempted God in their hearts. Psalm 78:18

4. God was angry with that generation, and he said, their hearts always go astray and they know not my ways. Hebrews 3:10

5. A man looking at a woman with lust has committed adultery with her in his heart. Matthew 5:28

6. They hardened their hearts. Hebrews 3:8

7. God allowed Moses to issue divorce certificates because of the people's hardness of heart. Matthew 19:8

8. Your eyes affect your heart. Lamentations 3:51

9. Be watchful lest your heart be taken in parties, drunkenness, and the cares of this world. Luke 21:34

10. The devil stole the word out of their hearts. Luke 8:12

11. The heart is deceitful above all things and desperately wicked. Who can know it? Jeremiah 17:9

12. The heart of the sons of men is full of evil, and madness is in their hearts while they live. Ecclesiastes 9:3

13. A gift destroys the heart. Ecclesiastes 7:7

19. DIVINE HEALTH

1. All over the world people are being healed by God from all kinds of sicknesses and diseases. Only believe.

2. Life and death are in the power of the tongue. And your words can be medicine or poison. So count your words.

3. Before medicating your kids or yourself with prescribed medicine for depression, ADD, etc., go to CCHR.org and see the dangers of psychiatry.

4. Like vaccines destroy diseases, so Christ destroyed death.

5. The years of your life will be many.

6. The thief comes only to steal, kill, and destroy.

7. The hearing ear and the seeing eye, the Lord made them both.

8. I will praise Him who is the health of my countenance. Thank God for your health and your healing.

9. Forgiving people often results in your healing and peace of mind.

10. Fear of a sickness acts as a magnet that negatively affects your health. But faith works like a repellent allowing working wonders.

11. The son of man manifested to destroy the works of the devil.

12. The Bible is full of people who were healed from contagious and cancerous diseases and even rose from the dead.

13. Elizabeth was barren. But her husband prayed until God answered his prayer and gave them a son who became a prophet.

14. I will take sickness from the midst of you.

15. He sent His Word and healed them.

19. DIVINE HEALTH

16. Jesus healed all sicknesses and cured all diseases, but he could do nothing for those who refused to come to him for healing.

17. He renews your youth like that of an eagle.

18. Curses and spells are canceled in the name of Jesus.

19. The leaves of the trees were for the healing of the nations.

20. Not all incurable diseases are fatal, but they are curable.

21. When God healed the waters, life flourished and there was no more death or bareness in it.

22. The servant knew a man of God who could heal her master.

23. He was sick near to death, but God had mercy on him.

24. Take a present to the man of God and ask of the Lord, 'Will I recover from this disease? And the king did recover.

25. For every disease there is an antidote.

26. Love mends hearts but bodies need medicine.

27. He went around doing good, healing all who were oppressed by the devil.

28. Lest they be converted, and I heal them indicates that some sickness is related to sin and disobedience.

29. Satan smote Job with boils, but the Lord healed him and added 140 years more to his life with happiness.

30. Oh Lord, spare me that I may recover strength.

31. God's health plan is for those who believe. By his stripes you are healed.

32. To you who fear My name will the son of righteousness arise with healing in His wings.

33. The body heals itself, but it is not the healer.

34. The sick came to Jesus, and they all went home healed.

35. Love healed more people than any known cure, and hate has killed more people than any known weapon.

36. Bless the Lord oh my soul and forget not all his benefits who forgives all my sins and heals me of all my diseases.

37. Pray for the sick and believe that they will recover in his name.

38. If you want to live forever, then eat from the tree of life. We die because Adam and Eve ate from the tree God said not to eat.

39. No matter how sick a society becomes, hope in God.

40. Jesus gave men the power to cast out demons and to heal all kinds of sicknesses and diseases in his name.

41. Doctors are instruments in God's health plan, and so are when you pray for the sick and lay your hands on them with or without a medical degree.

42. Life is in the blood. And so is sickness. Therefore do not eat meat with its blood.

43. Pleasant words will bring health to the bones.

44. Keep believing God for a cure and a miracle.

45. The word of God is life and medicine to all your flesh.

46. Healing is not always instantaneous, but it does start with the prayer of faith in Jesus name.

47. Hold your healing when God heals you less that sickness returns worse than before.

48. There is no medical cure for demonic ailments, but in Jesus name demons must leave a body when he is cast out leaving a person healed and in his right mind.

49. Pamper not the demons of chronic ailments, but shun them in Jesus' name and be healed.

50. A happy face shows a merry heart, but by sorrow of the heart the spirit is broken.

51. You look good when your soul looks better than your body.

52. An evil heart causes ailments that medicine cannot cure.

20. HEALING PROMISES

1. Go tell what things you have seen and heard: How the blind sees, the lame walk, the lepers are cleansed, the deaf hear, the dead are raised, and to the poor the Gospel is preached. Matthew 11:5

2. An evil disease, say they, cleave fast unto him. And now that he lies down he will rise up no more. Psalm 41:8

3. You will be blessed above all people. There will not be male or female barren among you, or your cattle. And the Lord will take away from you all sicknesses, and he will put none of the evil diseases of Egypt, which you know, on you, but will lay them on all of them that hate you. Deuteronomy 7:14

4. They will not say, I am sick. The people that dwell there will be forgiven for their iniquity. Isaiah 33:24

5. I will bring health and cure. And I will cure them and will reveal to them my abundance of peace and truth. Jeremiah 33:6

6. The Lord says: I will restore health to you, and heal you of all your wounds. Jeremiah 30:17

7. If my people who are called by my name will humble themselves and pray, and seek my face, and turn from their wicked ways, then I will hear from heaven, forgive their sin, and heal their land. 2 Chronicles 7:14

8. He sent his word and healed them and delivered them from their destruction. Psalm 107:20

9. I was dumb, I opened not my mouth, because you did it. Remove your stroke away from me. I am consumed by the blow of your hand. Psalm 39:9

10. Heal the sick, cleanse the lepers, raise the dead, and cast out

demons. Freely give as you have received. Matthew 10:8

11. The leaves of the tree are for the healing of the nations. Revelation 22:2

12. Jehovah (Rapha) will take away your illnesses and put none of the evil diseases of Egypt on you. Deuteronomy 7.:5

13. The Lord will strengthen you upon your sickbed. He will make your bed in your illnesses. Psalm 41:3

14. The Lord God is merciful, gracious, long-suffering, and abundant in goodness and truth. Exodus 34:6

15. He has seen your ways, and he will heal you. Isaiah 57:18

16. Fear not, only believe and you shall be made whole. Luke 8:50

17. And the blood will be to you for a token on the houses where you are. And when I see the blood, I will pass over you, and the plague will not be on you to destroy you when I smite the land of Egypt. Exodus 12:13

18. The Lord turned the captivity of Job when he prayed for his friends. Job 42:10

19. And in that day will the deaf hear the words of the book, and the eyes of the blind will see out of obscurity and out of the darkness. Isaiah 29:18

20. The light of the moon will be as the light of the sun, and the light of the sun will be 7 times as the light of 7 days, in the day that the Lord binds up the injuries of his people and heals the stroke of their wounds. Isaiah 30:26

21. He gives power to the faint and to those that have no might he increases strength. Even youths will faint and be weary, and the young men will utterly fall. But they that wait upon the Lord shall renew their strength. They will mount up with wings like eagles, they shall run and not be weary, and they will walk and not faint. Isaiah 30:29

22. Hear you deaf and look you blind, that you may see. Isaiah 42:18

23. Peter on this rock I will build my church, and the gates of

Hades will not prevail against it. I will give you the keys of the kingdom of heaven, and whatever you bind on earth will be bound in heaven, and whatever you lose on earth will be loosed in heaven. Matthew 16:18

24. I will not die but live to declare the works of the Lord. Psalm 118:17

25. We are raised up together and made to sit together in heavenly places in Christ Jesus. Ephesians 2:6

26. The weapons of your warfare are not carnal, but mighty through God to pull down strongholds and to cast down imaginations, and every high thing that exalts itself against the knowledge of God and to take captive every thought to be obedient to Christ. 2 Corinthians 10:4

27. You are precious in my sight and honorable and I have loved you. Therefore, will I give men for you, and people for your life. Isaiah 43:4

28. And I sought for a man among them, that should make up the hedge, and stand in the gap before Me for the land, that I should not destroy it, but I found none. Ezekiel 22:30

29. In a moment, in the twinkling of an eye, at the last trump, when the trumpet will sound, the dead will be raised incorruptible, and we will be changed. 1 Corinthians 15:52

30. So Abraham prayed to God. And God healed Abimelech, and his wife, and his maidservants; and they did bare children. Genesis 20:17

31. If you will diligently listen to the voice of the Lord God, and do that which is right in his sight, and give ear to his commandments and keep all his statutes, then will I put none of these diseases upon you which I have brought on the Egyptians. I am the Lord that heals you. Exodus 15:26

32. Give me life, so that I may praise You. Psalms 119:175

33. As Moses lifted up the serpent in the wilderness, even so must the son of man be lifted up, that whosoever believes in him should not perish, but have eternal life. John 3:14

34. You will walk in all the ways which the Lord God has commanded you, that you may live, and that it may be well with you, and that you may prolong your days in the land which you will possess. Deuteronomy 5:33

35. Bless the Lord, O my soul, and forget not all his benefits. Who forgives all my iniquities and who heals me of all my diseases. Psalm 103:1

36. And when the father of Publius became sick with a fever, and of a bloody flux, Paul went to him, and prayed, and laid his hands on him, and healed him. After this, many others on the island who had diseases came to him and were cured medically. Acts 28:7

37. There failed nothing, of any good thing, which the Lord had spoken to the house of Israel. It all came to pass. Joshua 21:45

38. And David built there an altar to the Lord and offered burnt offerings and peace offerings. So the Lord was entreated for the land, and the plague stayed from Israel. 1 Samuel 24:25

39. When heaven is shut up, and there is no rain because they have sinned against you. If they should pray toward this place, and confess your name, and turn from their sin when you afflicted them. Then hear in heaven and forgive the sin. 1 Kings 8:35

40. Blessed be the Lord, who has given rest to his people Israel, according to all that he has promised. There has not failed one word of all his good promises, which he promised by the hand of Moses his servant. 1 Kings 8:56

41. And Naaman the leper went down into the Jordan and dipped himself seven times according to the word of the man of God. And his skin became like that of a small child, and he was clean. Then he and the people with him returned to the man of God and he said to Elijah: Now I know that there is no God in all the earth, but in Israel. 2 Kings 5:14

42. Isaiah, go back and tell Hezekiah the captain of my people that the Lord says, I have heard your prayer, and I have seen your tears. I will heal you and add 15 more years to your life. And they

took a lump of figs as Isaiah said, and laid it on the boil, and he recovered. 2 Kings 20:5

43. He brought them out with silver and gold, and there was not one feeble person among them. Psalm 105:37

44. My Lord, God of Israel, there is no God like you in heaven nor in the earth that keeps covenant and shows mercy to your servants, that walk before you with all their hearts. 1 Chronicles 6:14

45. God is not a man, that he should lie. Neither the son of man, that he should repent. Has he said it, and will he not do it? Has he spoken, and will he not make it good? Numbers 23:19

46. The Lord listened to Hezekiah and healed the people. 2 Chronicles 30:20

47. Fasting God's way will cause your light to break forth as the morning, and your health spring forth quickly. Isaiah 58:8

48. Have mercy on me Lord and heal me. For I am weak, and my bones are vexed even my soul. Psalm 6:2

49. Many are the afflictions of the righteous, but the Lord delivers him out of them all. Psalm 34:19

50. The Lord will preserve you and keep you alive. He will be bless you on the earth. He will not deliver you to the will of your enemies. The Lord will strengthen you upon your bed of languishing. He will make your bed in sickness. Psalm 41:2

51. Why are you cast down my soul, and why so disquieted within? I will hope in God, and praise him, for he is the health of my countenance and my God. Psalm 42:11

52. That your way may be known on earth, your saving health among all nations. Psalm 67:2

53. Lord I cried to you, and you healed me. Psalm 30:2

54. Take balm for her pain, if so she may be healed. I would have healed her, but she is not healed. Jeremiah 51:8

55. My child, forget not my law, but let your heart keep my commandments. For length of days, long life, and peace, will they

add to you. Proverbs 3:1

56. My child, listen to my words and tune your ears to my sayings. Let them not depart from your eyes and keep them close to your heart. For they are life to those that find them and health to all their flesh. Keep your heart with all diligence, for out of it flows the issues of life. Proverbs 4:20

57. For by me your days will be multiplied, and the years of your life will be increased. Proverbs 9:11

58. They cried to the Lord in their trouble, and he saved them out of their distresses. He sent his word, healed and delivered them from their destruction. Oh, that men would praise the Lord for his goodness, and for his wonderful works to the children of men! Psalm 107:19

59. To you who fear my name, the sun of righteousness will arise with healing in his wings. Malachi 4:2

60. I am the Lord, the God of all flesh. Is there anything too hard for me? Jeremiah 32:27

61. Because you have made the Lord your refuge, and the Most High your habitation, no evil will befall you, neither will any plague come near your dwelling. And because you have loved me, will I deliver you and set you on high. And because you know my name, and call on me, will I answer you. I will be with you in trouble to deliver you and honor you, and with long life will I satisfy you, and show my salvation. Psalm 91

62. Are you sick? Let the elders of the church pray for you, anointing you with oil in the name of the Lord. And the prayer of faith will save the sick, and the Lord will raise him up. And if he has committed sins, they shall be forgiven him. Confess your faults one to another, and pray one for another, that you may be healed for the effectual fervent prayer of a righteous man avails much. James 5:14

63. By his stripes you are healed. Isaiah 53:5

64. Serve the Lord your God, and he will bless your bread and

water. He will take sickness away from the midst of you. Nothing will cast their young, or be barren in your land, and the number of your days he will fulfill. Exodus 23:25

65. If the Spirit of him that raised up Jesus from the dead dwells in you, he that raised Christ from the dead will also quicken your mortal bodies by his Spirit that dwells in you. Romans 8:11

66. Lord, if you are willing, you can make me clean. I will, be clean, Jesus responded. And immediately he was cleansed from his leprosy. Matthew 8:2

67. Go your way, as you have believed so will it be done to you. Matthew 8:13

68. He cast out evil spirits with his word and healed all that were sick. Matthew 8:16

69. When the crowd saw how Jesus healed the paralyzed man, they marveled and glorified God who had given such power unto men. Matthew 9:1

70. The healthy don't need a doctor, but the sick do. Matthew 9:12

71. Jesus, my child is dying, but come and lay your hands on her and she shall live. Matthew 9:18

72. Daughter be of good comfort. Your faith has made you whole. And the woman was made from that hour. Matthew 9:22

73. Jesus said to him, See, you have been made well. Go and sin no more lest a worse thing come on you. John 5:14

74. He will pray for you and you will live. Genesis 20:7

75. And Abraham was old, and well stricken in age, and the Lord had blessed Abraham in all things. Genesis 24:1

76. Women received their dead raised to life again. Hebrews 11:35

77. They have healed the hurt of the daughter of my people slightly, saying, Peace, peace, when there is no peace. Jeremiah 8:11

78. And many wonders and signs were done by the apostles. Acts 2:43

THE AUTHOR'S BOOKS

1. HEALING PROMISES: A Personal Guide to Health and Healing
2. SACRED AND PECULIAR: Poems For Young And Old
3. PARIS FRANCE MISSION: Stories And Prophecies
4. A PURE HEART: Biblical Truths On Love, Marriage, And Purity
5. QUOTES UNQUOTE: Thoughts On Life And Success
6. THE KING: Who Will Rule The World
7. PEACE LOVE WAR: 500 Reasons to Live or Die For
8. STARS, STRIPES, AND SECRETS: The Sins Of America
9. THE BOOK OF REVELATION: God Wants You To Know This Before The Apocalypse
10. MONEY TALKS: Stories Jesus Told The Rich And The Poor.
11. VUISBOEK: Die Stryd en Toekoms van God se Volk
12. PARIS MY LOVE - Ai Love Poems

Ebooks are free only on the website ParisFranceMission.org. If you love this content please share it with friends and family. Thank you for your love and support. Andre

THE END

www.ingramcontent.com/pod-product-compliance
Lightning Source LLC
Chambersburg PA
CBHW071102240526
45471CB00016B/2404